Cancer Bioinformatics

Edited by Ghedira Kais and Yosr Hamdi

Published in London, United Kingdom

Cancer Bioinformatics
http://dx.doi.org/10.5772/intechopen.94626
Edited by Ghedira Kais and Yosr Hamdi

Contributors
Arpana Parihar, Raju Khan, Shivani Malviya, Pavel Onofrei, Dragos Viorel Radu, Elena Carmen Cotrutz, Stoica Laura, Doinita Temelie-Olinici, Ana-Emanuela Botez, Vasile Bogdan Grecu, Alina-Alexandra Onofrei, Nicholas Nicholson, Francesco Giusti, Manola Bettio, Raquel Negrao Carvalho, Nadya Dimitrova, Tadeusz Dyba, Manuela Flego, Luciana Neamtiu, Giorgia Randi, Carmen Martos, Yelda A. Leal, Anwar Ebrahim, Ban Hussein Alwash, Rawan Asaad Jaber Al- Rubaye, Mustafa Mohammad Alaaraj, Donovan McGrowder, Lennox Anderson-Jackson, Lowell Dilworth, Shada Mohansingh, Melisa Anderson Cross, Sophia Bryan, Fabian Miller, Cameil Wilson-Clarke, Chukwuemeka Nwokocha, Ruby Alexander-Lindo, Shelly McFarlane, Ghedira Kais, Yosr Hamdi

Notice
Statements and opinions expressed in the chapters are these of the individual contributors and not necessarily those of the editors or publisher. No responsibility is accepted for the accuracy of information contained in the published chapters. The publisher assumes no responsibility for any damage or injury to persons or property arising out of the use of any materials, instructions, methods or ideas contained in the book.

First published in London, United Kingdom, 2022 by IntechOpen
IntechOpen is the global imprint of INTECHOPEN LIMITED, registered in England and Wales, registration number: 11086078, 5 Princes Gate Court, London, SW7 2QJ, United Kingdom
Printed in Croatia

British Library Cataloguing-in-Publication Data
A catalogue record for this book is available from the British Library

Additional hard and PDF copies can be obtained from orders@intechopen.com

Cancer Bioinformatics
Edited by Ghedira Kais and Yosr Hamdi
p. cm.

This title is part of the Biomedical Engineering Book Series, Volume 12
Topic: Bioinformatics and Medical Informatics
Series Editor: Robert Koprowski
Topic Editor: Slawomir Wilczynski

Print ISBN 978-1-83969-107-2
Online ISBN 978-1-83969-108-9
eBook (PDF) ISBN 978-1-83969-109-6
ISSN 2631-5343

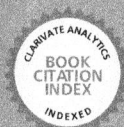

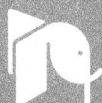

IntechOpen Book Series

Biomedical Engineering

Volume 12

Aims and Scope of the Series

Biomedical Engineering is one of the fastest-growing interdisciplinary branches of science and industry. The combination of electronics and computer science with biology and medicine has improved patient diagnosis, reduced rehabilitation time, and helped to facilitate a better quality of life. Nowadays, all medical imaging devices, medical instruments, or new laboratory techniques result from the cooperation of specialists in various fields. The series of Biomedical Engineering books covers such areas of knowledge as chemistry, physics, electronics, medicine, and biology. This series is intended for doctors, engineers, and scientists involved in biomedical engineering or those wanting to start working in this field.

Meet the Series Editor

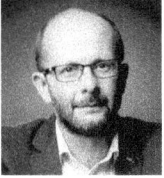

Robert Koprowski, MD (1997), Ph.D. (2003), Habilitation (2015), is an employee of the University of Silesia, Poland, Institute of Computer Science, Department of Biomedical Computer Systems. For 20 years, he has studied the analysis and processing of bio-medical images, emphasizing the full automation of measurement for a large inter-individual variability of patients. Dr. Koprowski has authored more than a hundred research papers with dozens in impact factor (IF) journals and has authored or co-authored six books. Additionally, he is the author of several national and international patents in the field of biomed-ical devices and imaging. Since 2011, he has been a reviewer of grants and projects (including EU projects) in biomedical engineering.

Meet the Volume Editors

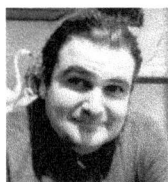

Kais Ghedira is a bioinformatician at Institut Pasteur de Tunis, Tunisia. He has been a principal investigator/co-investigator/WP leader for several national and international grants. He has contributed to building capacities in bioinformatics at the national and international levels. He is an active member of the Genome Tunisia Collaborative Alliance (GTCA) which aims to sequence Tunisian genomes to improve disease diagnostics in Tunisian patients. He is contributing to implementing genomic medicine in Tunisia, both the region and the continent. Dr. Ghedira is the author/co-author of more than fifty publications in highly ranked journals and is co-editor of several books. He is mainly interested in functional genomics, multiomics data integration, network generation and analysis, NGS data analysis, host-pathogen interaction study, and databases and webtools development.

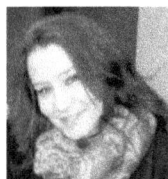

Yosr Hamdi is a biologist and researcher at Institut Pasteur de Tunis, Tunisia. She is a specialist in cancer genomics and precision oncology. Dr. Hamdi started in the field of human genetics in 2004 with the Human Genome Project. Then, she obtained a master's degree in Cellular and Molecular Biology at the Faculty of Medicine, Laval University, Canada. In 2009, she joined the Genomics Center of the Centre de Recherche du Centre Hospitalier de l'Université Laval (CRCHUL) where she obtained a Ph.D. in Molecular Medicine. Dr. Hamdi is now leading the Genome Tunisia Collaborative Alliance (GTCA) and the PerMediNA Consortium (Personalised Medicine in North Africa) to continue the investigations of cancer genomics in African populations as well as implement genomic medicine and precision oncology in North Africa.

Contents

Preface

Cancer Bioinformatics is organized around examples of the use of bioinformatics in precision oncology. It contains seven chapters.

Chapter 1 is an introductory chapter in which the editors introduce cancer as a complex and multifactorial disease and bioinformatics multiomics approaches that can be applied and used to study the disease.

Chapter 2, "Urologic Cancer Molecular Biology", focuses on molecular mechanisms underlying the urological carcinogenic processes, the molecular pathways involved in this process, and the biomarkers useful for diagnosis, predictability, and treatment to improve the outcomes of cancer patients.

Chapter 3, "Control of Cytoskeletal Dynamics in Cancer through a Combination of Cytoskeletal Components", investigates the molecular mechanism behind S100A4 function in epithelial-mesenchymal transition, demonstrating its participation in myosin dynamics modulation. Understanding the signaling pathways involved provides a better understanding of the changes that occur during metastasis leading to the identification of proteins that can be targeted for treatment, resulting in lower mortality.

Chapter 4, "Identification of Biomarkers Associated with Cancer Using Integrated Bioinformatic Analysis", reports various types of biomarkers associated with different types of cancer and their identification using integrated bioinformatic analysis. It also provides insight into integrated bioinformatics analysis tools and databases for cancer biomarkers prediction.

Chapter 5, "The Clinical Usefulness of Prostate Cancer Biomarkers: Current and Future Directions", reports emerging molecular biomarkers such as exosomal miRNAs and proteins that provide precise indications for cancer diagnostics, prognostics, and prediction and can be used in monitoring therapeutic response.

Chapter 6, "The Role of Registration in Cancer Control and Prevention", examines the importance of cancer registries that play an essential role in estimations of the burden of cancer for different geographic areas and in cancer control and prevention.

Chapter 7, "Dotting the "i" of Interoperability in FAIR Cancer-Registry Data Sets", describes an approach to making cancer registry data FAIR (findable, accessible, interoperable, and reusable) using ontologies with practical examples of how the validation rules can be modelled with description logic.

The editors would like to thank all the authors for their contributions. We are also grateful to IntechOpen, particularly Ms. Maja Bozicevic and Ms. Anja Filipovic, for their assistance and patience throughout the publication process of this book.

Ghedira Kais
Laboratory of Bioinformatics, Biomathematics and Biostatistics,
Institut Pasteur de Tunis,
Université Tunis El Manar,
Tunis, Tunisia

Yosr Hamdi
Laboratory of Biomedical Genomics and Oncogenetics,
Institut Pasteur de Tunis,
Université Tunis El Manar,
Tunis, Tunisia

Section 1

Bioinformatics Applications to Identify Molecular Mechanisms, Pathways and Biomarkers in Cancers

Chapter 1

Introductory Chapter: Application of Bioinformatics Tools in Cancer Prevention, Screening, and Diagnosis

Ghedira Kais and Yosr Hamdi

1. Introduction

Cancer is a leading cause of death worldwide, with nearly 10 million deaths in 2020, accounting for one in six deaths. Breast, lung, colon rectum, and prostate are considered the most common cancer types [1]. Around one-third of deaths from cancer are due to environmental factors and lifestyle habits, such as tobacco use, high body mass index, alcohol consumption, low fruit and vegetable intake, and lack of physical activity [2]. In addition, 10% of cancer cases are due to genetic factors and around 10% of cancer-causing infections, such as human papillomavirus (HPV) and hepatitis, are responsible for approximately 30% of cancer cases in low- and lower-middle-income countries [3]. Indeed, HPV infection is the main cause of cervical cancer, cancer that can be cured if detected early and treated effectively [4]. The multifactorial character of the disease with the huge amount of data that has been generated during the last decades covering all risk factors behind cancer disease allowed bioinformatics to play an essential role in Cancer research and made oncology a success story in translating and using OMICs data, including genomics, transcriptomics and proteomics data, in clinical settings [5].

2. Use of bioinformatics integrative approaches in oncology

Numerous research groups worldwide have attempted to develop strategies to identify novel diagnostic and prognostic markers for different cancer types based on computational integrative analyzes and tools. One of the most powerful computational approaches is meta-analysis, where multiple studies interrogating a common hypothesis are analyzed together [6]. Several studies have applied meta-analysis methods to cancer microarray data in order to identify differentially expressed genes (DEGs) between cancer patients and controls. These methods can be applied to identify robust gene-expression signatures in a single cancer type and/or to look for common expression patterns across different types of cancer. In 2004, Rhodes and co-workers investigated and analyzed 40 published cancer microarray data sets, comprising 38 million gene expression measurements from >3700 cancer samples [7]. With the advent of high throughput sequencing technology, known as NGS,

RNA sequencing (RNASeq) has been used in several aspects of cancer research and therapy including the discovery of biomarkers, the characterization of cancer heterogeneity and evolution, cancer immunotherapy, and the investigation of drug resistance [8]. High throughput sequencing technology has the advantage of fast-speed sequencing at low cost and with high accuracy compared to the former Sanger technology. Compared to microarray, RNASeq can also detect unknown gene expression sequences [9]. Gene expression profiling often generates large gene-expression signatures that need to be functionally analyzed to identify a handful of genes of interest that are selected for experimental validation. Several methods have been developed allowing systematic functional analysis of gene expression signatures including Gene Ontology (GO) [10, 11], KEGG [12], TransPath [13], and GenMAPP [14]. Finally, to better understand complex biological processes, such as cancer initiation and progression, it is important to consider the integration of transcriptomic data in the context of complex molecular networks. This implies the mapping of interactomes involving protein-protein interaction with the gene expression signature to identify induced or repressed interactome subnetworks on the basis of known and predicted protein-protein interactions [15].

3. Data science in oncology

In the past decade, Artificial intelligence (AI), particularly, machine learning (ML) has grown rapidly in the context of data analysis and computing allowing applications and platforms to function in an intelligent manner (https://pubmed.ncbi.nlm.nih.gov/34278328/). ML is a field that refers to a broad range of learning algorithms that perform intelligent predictions based on learning from a subset of data [16]. AI has recently altered the landscape of cancer research and medical oncology using traditional ML algorithms and cutting-edge Deep Learning (DL) approaches [17]. Indeed, ML algorithms including Random Forest (RF), Gradient Boosting Machine (GBM), and Neural Network (NN) have been used to optimize cancer classification [18]. Furthermore, DL-based algorithms have been widely applied in medical imaging to accurately diagnose breast cancer [19], colorectal cancer [20], lung cancer [21], and others [22]. Moreover, AI systems have been developed and used to diagnose early gastric cancer (EGC) from 4667 magnifying image-enhanced endoscopy images, including 1950 EGC images from 1042 cases and 2717 noncancerous images from 769 cases [23].

4. Tools and databases

Several publicly accessible databases containing cancer related data, and integrating tools for delivering and analyzing information and data, as well as specialized databases dedicated to specific types of cancer, have been developed during the last decades. Most commonly used and prominent ones include the International Cancer Genome Consortium (ICGC) [24] and The Cancer Genome Atlas (TCGA) [25]. A detailed list of publicly available databases and their descriptions has been reported by Pavlopoulou and co-workers [26]. Recently, a novel database integrating RNA-seq, DNA methylation, and related clinical data from over 10,000 cancer patients in the TCGA study as well as from normal tissues in the GTEx study has been developed and made freely available through [27, 28]. Concerning bioinformatics and computational tools for cancer risk prediction, numerous resources have been developed including the International Breast Cancer Intervention Study (IBIS) [29], the Breast and Ovarian Analysis of Disease Incidence and Carrier Estimation Algorithm (BOADICEA) [30], the BRCAPRO [31] and the Breast Cancer Surveillance Consortium (BCSC) risk model [32]. A comprehensive list of web tools and web servers for cancer genomic study and cancer prognosis analysis has been provided by Yang and coworkers [33] and Zheng and colleagues [34].

5. Precision oncology application

Molecular and genetic profiling of tumors play an increasingly important role not only in cancer research but also in the clinical management of cancer patients [35]. Multi-omics approaches hold the promise of improving diagnostics, prognostics, and personalized treatment using highly reproducible and robust bioinformatics methods of complex data management and integration to go from the primary analysis of raw molecular profiling data to the automatic generation of a clinical report and its delivery to decision-making clinical oncologists [36]. The initial results coming out from these efforts are promising, but it has also become explicit that the exploitation of the full potential of precision oncology faces many challenges. One major bottleneck resides in the efficient and precise annotation of variants [37]. This challenge requires the use of databases containing well-curated variants as well as their interactions with potential drugs. The second challenge is the rapid development of molecular profiling techniques coming with novel challenges in terms of the development of new bioinformatics tools, pipelines, and workflows adapted to each of these new techniques [38]. Moreover, multi-omics approaches are providing more insights into dysregulated pathways, increasing the level of confidence in reporting actionable variants when they can be confirmed by RNA, protein, or epigenetic profiling. However, the availability of diverse multi-omics data is currently posing new bioinformatics challenges to integrate multiple data sets and identifying potentially efficient treatments [39]. Finally, interpreting the clinical significance of genomic variants and transcriptional changes is a laborious task that cannot be fully automated in a reliable way and therefore needs a multidisciplinary team to apply clinical interpretation to select relevant variants and to recommend targeted, personalized therapies [40]. That being said, bioinformatics still holds the hope to make the intersection of cancer research and medical applications for better clinical management of patients.

Author details

Ghedira Kais[1]* and Yosr Hamdi[2]*

1 Laboratory of Bioinformatics, Biomathematics and Biostatistics, Institut Pasteur de Tunis, Université Tunis El Manar, Tunis, Tunisia

2 Laboratory of Biomedical Genomics and Oncogenetics, Institut Pasteur de Tunis, Université Tunis El Manar, Tunis, Tunisia

*Address all correspondence to: ghedirakais@gmail.com
and yosr.hamdi@pasteur.utm.tn

IntechOpen

References

[1] Ferlay J, Ervik M, Lam F, Colombet M, Mery L, Piñeros M, et al. Global Cancer Observatory: Cancer Today. Lyon: International Agency for Research on Cancer; 2020

[2] Cancer Prevention Overview (PDQ®)–Patient Version was originally published by the National Cancer Institute

[3] de Martel C, Georges D, Bray F, Ferlay J, Clifford GM. Global burden of cancer attributable to infections in 2018: A worldwide incidence analysis. The Lancet Global Health. 2020;**8**(2): e180-e190

[4] Burd EM. Human papillomavirus and cervical cancer. Clinical Microbiology Reviews. 2003;**16**(1):1-17. DOI: 10.1128/ CMR.16.1.1-17.2003

[5] Brenner C. Applications of bioinformatics in Cancer. Cancers (Basel). 2019;**11**(11):1630. DOI: 10.3390/ cancers11111630

[6] Rhodes D, Chinnaiyan A. Integrative analysis of the cancer transcriptome. Nature Genetics. 2005;**37**:S31-S37. DOI: 10.1038/ng1570

[7] Rhodes DR, Yu J, Shanker K, et al. Large-scale meta-analysis of cancer microarray data identifies common transcriptional profiles of neoplastic transformation and progression. Proceedings of the National Academy of Sciences of the United States of America. 2004;**101**(25):9309-9314. DOI: 10.1073/ pnas.0401994101

[8] Wang Y, Mashock M, Tong Z, Mu X, Chen H, Zhou X, et al. Changing technologies of RNA sequencing and their applications in clinical oncology.

Frontiers in Oncology. 2020;**10**:447. DOI: 10.3389/fonc.2020.00447

[9] Marioni JC, Mason CE, Mane SM, Stephens M, Gilad Y. RNA-seq: An assessment of technical reproducibility and comparison with gene expression arrays. Genome Research. 2008;**18**(9): 1509-1517. DOI: 10.1101/gr.079558.108

[10] Harris MA, Clark J, Ireland A, Lomax J, Ashburner M, Foulger R, et al. The gene ontology (GO) database and informatics resource. Nucleic Acids Research. 2004;**32**(Database issue): D258-D261. DOI: 10.1093/nar/gkh036

[11] Draghici S, Khatri P, Bhavsar P, Shah A, Krawetz SA, Tainsky MA. Onto-tools, the toolkit of the modern biologist: Onto-express, onto-compare, onto-design and onto-translate. Nucleic Acids Research. 2003;**31**(13):3775-3378. DOI: 10.1093/nar/gkg624

[12] Kanehisa M, Furumichi M, Sato Y, Ishiguro-Watanabe M, Tanabe M. KEGG: Integrating viruses and cellular organisms. Nucleic Acids Research. 2021;**49**(D1):D545-D551. DOI: 10.1093/ nar/gkaa970

[13] Krull M, Voss N, Choi C, Pistor S, Potapov A, Wingender E. TRANSPATH: An integrated database on signal transduction and a tool for array analysis. Nucleic Acids Research. 2003;**31**(1): 97-100. DOI: 10.1093/nar/gkg089

[14] Doniger SW, Salomonis N, Dahlquist KD, et al. MAPPFinder: Using gene ontology and GenMAPP to create a global gene-expression profile from microarray data. Genome Biology. 2003;**4**:R7. DOI: 10.1186/gb-2003-4-1-r7

[15] Erdogan F, Radu TB, Orlova A, Qadree AK, de Araujo ED, Israelian J,

et al. JAK-STAT core cancer pathway: An integrative cancer interactome analysis. Journal of Cellular and Molecular Medicine. 2022;**26**(7):2049-2062. DOI: 10.1111/jcmm.17228. Epub 2022 Mar 1. PMID: 35229974; PMCID: PMC8980946

[16] Choi RY, Coyner AS, Kalpathy-Cramer J, Chiang MF, Campbell JP. Introduction to machine learning, neural networks, and deep learning. Translational Vision Science & Technology. 2020;**9**(2):14. DOI: 10.1167/tvst.9.2.14

[17] Kourou K, Exarchos KP, Papaloukas C, Sakaloglou P, Exarchos T, Fotiadis DI. Applied machine learning in cancer research: A systematic review for patient diagnosis, classification and prognosis. Computational and Structural Biotechnology Journal. 2021;**19**:5546-5555. DOI: 10.1016/j.csbj.2021.10.006

[18] Ramroach S, Joshi A, John M. Optimisation of cancer classification by machine learning generates an enriched list of candidate drug targets and biomarkers. Molecular Omics. 2020;**16**(2):113-125. DOI: 10.1039/c9mo00198k

[19] Shang LW, Ma DY, Fu JJ, Lu YF, Zhao Y, Xu XY, et al. Fluorescence imaging and Raman spectroscopy applied for the accurate diagnosis of breast cancer with deep learning algorithms. Biomedical Optics Express. 2020;**11**(7):3673-3683. DOI: 10.1364/BOE.394772

[20] Choi K, Choi SJ, Kim ES. Computer-aided Diagonosis for colorectal Cancer using deep learning with visual explanations. Annual International Conference of the IEEE Engineering in Medicine & Biology Society. 2020;**2020**:1156-1159. DOI: 10.1109/EMBC44109.2020.9176653

[21] Shimazaki A, Ueda D, Choppin A, Yamamoto A, Honjo T, Shimahara Y, et al. Deep learning-based algorithm for lung cancer detection on chest radiographs using the segmentation method. Scientific Reports. 2022;**12**(1): 727. DOI: 10.1038/s41598-021-04667-w

[22] Ma CY, Zhou JY, Xu XT, Guo J, Han MF, Gao YZ, et al. Deep learning-based auto-segmentation of clinical target volumes for radiotherapy treatment of cervical cancer. Journal of Applied Clinical Medical Physics. 2022;**23**(2):e13470. DOI: 10.1002/acm2.13470

[23] Abe S, Tomizawa Y, Saito Y. Can artificial intelligence be your angel to diagnose early gastric cancer in real clinical practice? Gastrointestinal Endoscopy. 2022;**95**(4):679-681. DOI: 10.1016/j.gie.2021.12.042

[24] International Cancer Genome Consortium, Hudson TJ, Anderson W, Artez A, Barker AD, et al. International network of cancer genome projects. Nature. 2010;**464**(7291):993-998. DOI: 10.1038/nature08987

[25] Cancer Genome Atlas Research Network, Weinstein JN, Collisson EA, Mills GB, Shaw KR, Ozenberger BA, et al. The Cancer genome atlas Pan-Cancer analysis project. Nature Genetics. 2013;**45**(10):1113-1120. DOI: 10.1038/ng.2764

[26] Pavlopoulou A, Spandidos DA, Michalopoulos I. Human cancer databases (review). Oncology Reports. 2015;**33**(1):3-18. DOI: 10.3892/or.2014.3579

[27] Tang G, Cho M, Wang X. OncoDB: An interactive online database for analysis of gene expression and viral infection in cancer. Nucleic Acids Research. 2022;**50**(D1):D1334-D1339. DOI: 10.1093/nar/gkab970

[28] Tang G, Cho M, Wang X. OncoDB: An interactive online database for analysis of gene expression and viral infection in cancer. Nucleic Acids Research. 2022;**50**(D1):D1334-D1339

[29] Tyrer J, Duffy SW, Cuzick J. A breast cancer prediction model incorporating familial and personal risk factors. Statistics in Medicine. 2004;**23**(7):1111-1130. DOI: 10.1002/sim.1668. Erratum in: Statistics in Medicine 2005 Jan 15;24(1):156

[30] Lee A, Mavaddat N, Wilcox AN, Cunningham AP, Carver T, Hartley S, et al. BOADICEA: A comprehensive breast cancer risk prediction model incorporating genetic and nongenetic risk factors. Genetics in Medicine. 2019;**21**(8):1708-1718. DOI: 10.1038/s41436-018-0406-9

[31] Antoniou AC, Hardy R, Walker L, Evans DG, Shenton A, Eeles R, et al. Predicting the likelihood of carrying a BRCA1 or BRCA2 mutation: Validation of BOADICEA, BRCAPRO, IBIS, myriad and the Manchester scoring system using data from UK genetics clinics. Journal of Medical Genetics. 2008;**45**(7):425-431. DOI: 10.1136/jmg.2007.056556

[32] Shieh Y, Hu D, Ma L, Huntsman S, Gard CC, Leung JW, et al. Breast cancer risk prediction using a clinical risk model and polygenic risk score. Breast Cancer Research and Treatment. 2016;**159**(3): 513-525. DOI: 10.1007/s10549-016-3953-2

[33] Yang Y, Dong X, Xie B, Ding N, Chen J, Li Y, et al. Databases and web tools for cancer genomics study. Genomics Proteomics Bioinformatics. 2015;**13**(1):46-50. DOI: 10.1016/j. gpb.2015.01.005. [Epub 2015 Feb 21]. Erratum in: Genomics Proteomics Bioinformatics. 2015 Jun;13(3):202-203

[34] Zheng H, Zhang G, Zhang L, et al. Comprehensive review of web servers and bioinformatics tools for Cancer prognosis analysis. Frontiers in Oncology. 2020;**10**:68. DOI: 10.3389/fonc.2020.00068

[35] Dietel M, Jöhrens K, Laffert MV, Hummel M, Bläker H, Pfitzner BM, et al. A 2015 update on predictive molecular pathology and its role in targeted cancer therapy: A review focussing on clinical relevance. Cancer Gene Therapy. 2015;**22**(9):417-430. DOI: 10.1038/cgt.2015.39

[36] Orlov YL, Baranova AV, Tatarinova TV. Bioinformatics methods in medical genetics and genomics. International Journal of Molecular Sciences. 2020;**21**(17):6224. DOI: 10.3390/ijms21176224

[37] Fröhlich H, Balling R, Beerenwinkel N, et al. From hype to reality: Data science enabling personalized medicine. BMC Medicine. 2018;**16**(1):150. DOI: 10.1186/s12916-018-1122-7

[38] Singer J, Irmisch A, Ruscheweyh HJ, et al. Bioinformatics for precision oncology. Briefings in Bioinformatics. 2019;**20**(3):778-788. DOI: 10.1093/bib/bbx143

[39] Miller DT, Lee K, Gordon AS, Amendola LM, Adelman K, Bale SJ, et al. ACMG secondary findings working group. Recommendations for reporting of secondary findings in clinical exome and genome sequencing, 2021 update: A policy statement of the American College of Medical Genetics and Genomics (ACMG). Genetics in Medicine. 2021;**23**(8):1391-1398. DOI: 10.1038/s41436-021-01171-4

[40] Qian M, Li Q, Zhang M, et al. Multidisciplinary therapy strategy of precision medicine in clinical practice. Clinical and Translational Medicine. 2020;**10**(1):116-124. DOI: 10.1002/ctm2.15

Chapter 2

Urologic Cancer Molecular Biology

Pavel Onofrei, Viorel Dragoș Radu, Alina-Alexandra Onofrei,
Stoica Laura, Doinita Temelie-Olinici, Ana-Emanuela Botez,
Vasile Bogdan Grecu and Elena Carmen Cotrutz

Abstract

An adequate understanding of the molecular mechanisms of the most common urological cancers is necessary for a correct approach to diagnosis, precise treatment, but also for the follow-up of these patients. It is necessary to understand the molecular mechanisms underlying the carcinogenic processes, the molecular pathways involved in this process, and also to describe the biomarkers useful for diagnosis but also for predictability, treatment, and natural history. In addition, it would be useful to describe a list of useful molecules currently under investigation as possible biomarkers to improve the income of cancer patients.

Keywords: prostate cancer, urothelial cancer, kidney cancer, biomarkers, bioinformatics

1. Introduction

Over the past decades, the treatment of localized cancers was mostly focused on surgery and radiotherapy and advanced neoplasia was treated using nonspecific cytotoxic agents. Despite the increasing 5-year survival rate, there is also still a large number of nonresponsive patients, mostly due to the diversity of genetic profiles among the worldwide population, also the heterogeneity within the tumor itself [1–3].

Neoplasia develops under a various number of molecular and genetic malfunctions that regulate cell division, cell differentiation, and programmed cell death [4, 5]. Tumor suppressor genes and proteins encoded by these genes play a major role in cellular growth regulation, cell signaling, and DNA repair. Oncogenes are mutated forms of normal genes and are associated with cellular proliferation.

Molecular biology focuses on the study of physiological and pathological changes in the body. It helps to develop tools for early diagnosis of these changes and ways to reverse them. In recent years, considerable efforts have been made to elucidate the molecular mechanisms of malignant transformation that have the role of personalized medicine (especially oncology) in order to maximize the effectiveness of the therapeutic response but also to minimize side effects. In this sense, understanding the process of carcinogenesis helps to diagnose at an early stage, an accurate diagnosis but also of the different behavior of tumor subtypes, in order to establish the appropriate therapy [6–11].

IntechOpen

BCG (Calmette-Guérin bacillus) immunological therapy in the treatment of bladder cancer is an excellent starting point for the usefulness of molecular studies on immunotherapy in genitourinary cancers. Being a nonspecific agent, there are many gaps regarding its mechanism of action but it paved the way for a different approach, that of inducing an immune response against cancer via cancer vaccines. Prostate and kidney cancer are also considered for this kind of treatment [11].

From a clinical point of view, the most obvious mechanism is the limitation of the specific antigen immune response by CD4 and CD8 (tumor-infiltrating lymphocytes) with significant importance in limiting the antitumor response thus preventing a significant proportion the clinical remission of tumors. Thus, a therapeutic line has been developed that targets an immune checkpoint blockade in order to bypass the mechanisms that limit the response, and which in the case of bladder tumors, in combination with conventional chemotherapy, or VEGF inhibition (vascular endothelial growth factor) in kidney cancer and last but not least, in prostate cancer—hormone therapy, increase the effectiveness of treatment [11].

In this chapter, we discuss the most significant urological cancers including prostate cancer, urothelial carcinoma, and renal highlighting their molecular mechanisms and the related studied biomarkers for precision diagnosis and therapeutic management.

1.1 Bioinformatics in urologic cancers

Cancer is one of the most complex diseases to understand. It is characterized by the rapid growth and spread of its cells, its resistance to conventional treatments, and its ability to invade and displace normal tissue. Malignant cells, regardless of type, usually share some common features—reprogrammed energy metabolism, sustained cell growth signals, evasion of growth suppressors, resistance to apoptosis, facilitation of replicative immortality, induction of angiogenesis, resistance to destruction by the immune system, and promotion of cell invasion and metastasis. These recognized characteristics have led to a deeper understanding of this disease. However, the reality is that our overall ability to cure cancer has not yet improved significantly, especially for adult cancers, which account for 99% of all cancers [12–14].

The major challenges facing clinical oncologists include not only the considerable heterogeneity and different genetic backgrounds even within the same type of cancer, but also the fact that effective drugs lose their efficacy due to the ability of cancer to evolve rapidly, especially with regard to the emergence of drug-resistant subpopulations [12–14].

One of the many reasons why our knowledge is so sparse is the lack of molecular-level data, the full analysis, and interpretation of which can reveal the full complexity of developing cancer. Although large amounts of genomic, epigenomic, transcriptomic, metabolomic, and proteomic data have been obtained for a variety of cancers, few cancer studies are designed to fully exploit all the information that can be derived from the available omic data [12–14]. Integrative analyses of multiple data types may prove to be essential to gain a full and systems-level understanding of cancer's evolution dynamics, including the elucidation of its true drivers as well as key facilitators at different developmental stages of cancer. We anticipate that only when all of the key information hidden in omic data can be fully derived and utilized can we expect a meaningful breakthrough in our understanding of cancer [12–14].

The understanding of the human genome combined with technologies such as DNA and protein arrays or mass spectrometry has improved the simultaneous study of numerous genes and proteins in single experiments and has rekindled interest in the search for novel biomarkers for cancers such as but not limited to, renal, urothelial, and prostate cancers [15–21]. Modern technology allows for parallel studies as compared to the serial analyses used in older methods. This allows the identification of distinct patterns for cancer diagnosis and classification, as well as for prediction of therapeutic response. In addition, these technologies enable the discovery of new individual tumor markers through the use of acceptable hypotheses and novel analytical methods [15–21]. Although new technologies and tactics often fail in the discovery of established cancer biomarkers and focus on identifying high-incidence compounds, they have the potential to revolutionize biomarker discovery. It is now critical to focus on thorough validation studies to discover the most effective techniques and biomarkers and bring them to the clinic as quickly as possible [15–21].

Bioinformatics and computational techniques have been well applied in the studies of various tumors (urologic, digestive gynecologic, etc.), and confirmed to be efficient and reliable in identifying novel tumor markers for cancer diagnosis and targeted treatments [22].

The very large pool of publicly available cancer-omic data, which includes transcriptomic, genomic, metabolomic, and epigenomic data, contains a considerable amount of information about the activities of individual biochemical pathways, their dynamics, and the complex relationships between them, as well as information about various microenvironmental factors. When the right questions are asked, powerful statistical analysis techniques can be very helpful in uncovering such information. Such targeted questions provide a framework for hypothesis-driven data analysis and evaluation that can be used to test the validity of the formulated hypothesis and to formulate new questions that may lead to the discovery of specific pathways or even possible causal relationships between the activities of different pathways. More effective analysis methods for different omic data formats are definitely needed to answer more difficult and in-depth questions about the data, such as deconvolution of gene expression data obtained from tissue samples with different cell types and inference of causal relationships. Effective data mining and information discovery require integrative analysis of various forms of omic and computational data [14, 15, 17–21].

1.2 Prostate cancer (PCa)

It is considered the second most prevalent cancer among male subjects. Around one in eight men will get diagnosed with the illness during their lifetime. In 2012, around 1.1 million men were diagnosed with prostate cancer globally. Around one in 40 of them will die due to this disease [23–25].

With the discovery and introduction of PSA-based screening tests, the incidence of prostate cancer has increased dramatically. However, given the advances in molecular biology, we realize that a purely PSA-based test does not provide sufficient accuracy. To find an answer, we need to consider other possible screening methods by elucidating the molecular basis of cancer development and more specific biomarkers [23–25].

The complexity of the diagnostic process in prostate cancer is reflected in the various interactions that occur during the course of the disease itself. The initial changes that lead to cancer are usually caused by chronic inflammation and dietary habits. They eventually lead to severe damage to the DNA of the prostate cells. Early genetic events that can promote disease progression include fusions or mutations of various genes and oncogenes (**Figure 1**), as well as malfunctions of molecular signaling pathways [23–25].

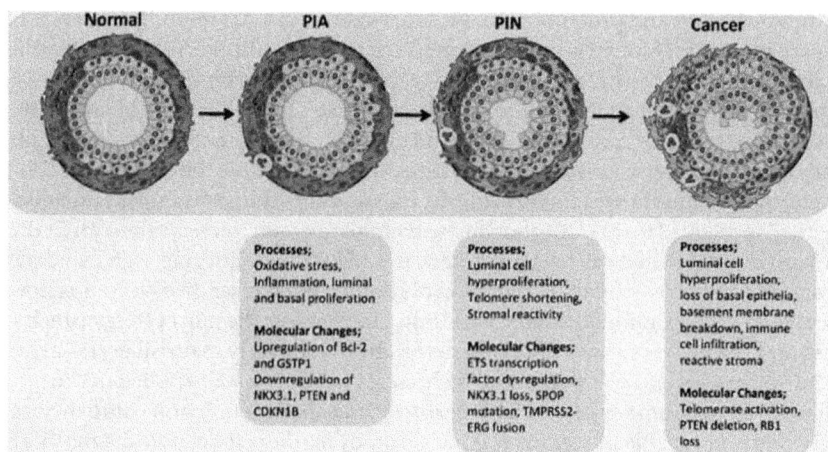

Figure 1.
Alterations that occur in the malignancy of prostatic tissue. PIA - proliferative inflammatory atrophy, PIN - prostatic intraepithelial neoplasia.

The primary androgen of the prostate is dihydrotestosterone (DHT), and exposure to this androgen is considered to be a precipitating factor in the development of primary prostatic neoplasia. The androgen receptor (AR) plays a central role in the development and progression of prostate cancer. Although the relationship between androgen exposure and cancer is not yet clear, exposure to very high or low concentrations of this substance may be protective against PCa (prostate cancer). The effects of androgen on long-term male survival are still unknown. The interaction of vitamin D with its receptor may influence the aggressiveness of the disease and its risk factors, but the mechanism underlying this event is not yet fully understood [23–25].

The prostate develops just caudal to the bladder neck by the proliferation of epithelial buds growing from the urogenital sinus epithelium. Epithelial budding is strictly androgen-dependent and represents the first identifiable events in prostate development. Budding of the prostate requires complicated epithelial-mesenchymal interactions [26, 27].

High testosterone levels in male embryos promote prostate development. Testosterone is converted to DHT by 5α-reductase, an interaction that activates AR. High testosterone levels during early development led to prostate growth regardless of genetic sex, suggesting a primary role for androgens in prostate induction [26, 27].

The upregulation of Sox9 (sex-determining region Y-box 9), a transcription factor induced by the FGF pathway, is the earliest event that appears to occur in the epithelium during prostate development. This mechanism is followed by the increased expression of Nkx3.1 (NK homeobox transcription family member), which influences the degree of branching in the mature mouse prostate, where it may also act as a tumor suppressor [26, 27].

The FGF family of secreted peptides promotes cell growth by binding to cell surface proteins and activating multiple signaling cascades demonstrated for prostate, mammary and salivary glands, or lung. Fgf-7 (keratinocyte growth factor) and Fgf-10 are considered specific for the prostate [28, 29]. Fgf-7 (keratinocyte growth factor) and Fgf-10 are considered specific for the prostate. FGFR2 is expressed in developing prostatic epithelial cells (PrECs) and through interaction with Frs-2α. Both molecules are secreted by the mesenchyme of the prostate. This mechanism led to the hypothesis that they act as andromedins since they are associated with androgen-independent growth factors. Due to the absence of Fgf-10, the mice also showed prostatic hypoplasia [28, 29].

Wnt signaling plays a crucial role in the development of various organs, including the prostate. Essentially, it regulates proliferation and differentiation through a series of Wnt ligands expressed during prostate bud formation. Canonical Wnt targets, such as Lef1 and Axin2, are upregulated in prostate bud epithelium [30–32].

Prostate cancer is one of the few malignancies for which there is a clinically meaningful serum biomarker. From its discovery in 1979 to its clinical application in the late 1980s to 1990s, PSA has become an invaluable tool for detecting, grading, and monitoring prostate cancer in men.

There is also considerable overlap in serum PSA levels between men with cancer and those with the noncancerous disease. The presence of prostatic hyperplasia or inflammation may also explain the elevated serum PSA levels [33, 34]. To this end, the use of PSA derivatives such as PSA density, PSA velocity, age-adjusted values, and more recently molecular derivatives can be used to improve clinical decisions compared to the isolated use of PSA.

Several molecular approaches have been pursued in the search for the optimal biomarker for prostate cancer. An overview of basic cellular processes begins with a DNA sequence (gene) that is transcribed into mRNA (transcript) and then translated into a protein that can then perform a specific cellular function. A major goal of biomarker development is to identify the differences in the molecular structure of prostate cancer cells compared to their benign counterparts and also to distinguish the more aggressive phenotypes from the others. The identification and quantification of these molecular differences in tissues and body fluids form the basis for the discovery of biomarkers for prostate cancer.

PSMA (glycoprotein prostate-specific membrane antigen), a folate hydrolase, has been studied as a potential biomarker for prostate cancer in tissue, serum, or urine. It is found in the membrane of all prostate epithelial cells. It is a type II transmembrane protein with an extracellular C-terminus that exists as a dimer and binds glutamate and glutamate-like structures [35, 36]. Nowadays, PSMA is mainly used in targeted imaging and theranostics [37, 38]. In particular, 68Gallium positron emission tomography of prostate-specific membrane antigen (68Ga-PSMA PET) is increasingly used as a diagnostic tool in biochemical recurrence after primary therapy [39].

Human kallikrein peptidase 2 (hK2) shares many important properties with PSA and has demonstrated its potential as another tumor marker for prostate cancer. Among many other similarities, hK2 and PSA share 80% amino acid homology, show similar specificity for prostate tissue, and are hormonally regulated by androgens. One of the major functions of hK2 is to activate the zymogen (proPSA) to active PSA by cleaving the amino acid presequence. Critical to its utility as a biomarker is that hK2 expression varies independently of tissue and serum PSA expression. In BPH, PSA expression is highly expressed compared to the minimal immunoreactivity of hK2, but hK2 is also overexpressed in PCa compared to PSA. Furthermore, tissue expression of hK2 appears to correlate with more aggressive pathological features, including Gleason grade [40, 41].

Circulating tumor cells (CTCs) have long been touted as potential prognostic biomarkers and indicators of treatment response. Subsequent CTC research in prostate cancer has employed a wide range of methods utilizing characteristics such as size, surface marker expression, and cellular plasticity that distinguish CTCs from circulating blood mononuclear cells [42, 43]. Typically, CTCs are defined as

CD45 and positive for an epithelial marker such as epithelial cell adhesion molecule (EpCAM) and/or cytokeratin. Although the development of CTCs as biomarkers for prostate cancer has been relatively slow, there has been considerable recent progress in the field and a growing number of clinical trials. Currently, there is only one FDA-approved method for identifying CTCs: CellSearch, which uses antibodies to EpCAM for CTC detection and then stains with antibodies to CD45 and cytokeratins 8, 18, and 19 (positive) to identify individual CTCs. Using this system, a CTC count of five or more cells per 7.5 mL of blood at any time during disease progression has been associated with poor prognosis in the prostate, breast, and colorectal cancers [42, 43].

The ease of collection of urine and the excretion of prostate cells have long made it a potential biomarker source for the early detection of prostate cancer [44]. However, only recently have urine biomarkers for prostate cancer come into clinical use. The first of these biomarkers, described in 1999, prostate cancer antigen 3 (PCA3), is not expressed outside the prostate. Studies show that PCA3 levels in prostate cancer are far higher than those in BPH, but the function of the antigen is still unknown [45, 46]. Recent studies used RT-PCR to detect PCA3 in urine and showed that PCA3 performs better than PSA in diagnosing PCa [47, 48].

Annexin A3 is a protein that is being studied as a possible biomarker for prostate cancer in urine. It belongs to a family of proteins known as phospholipid-binding proteins and shows altered expression in PCa [49].

α-Methylacyl coenzyme A racemase (AMACR) is an enzyme responsible for beta-oxidation of branched-chain fatty acids found in a diet consisting of beef and dairy products. Recent studies have shown that 88% of prostate carcinomas, as well as untreated metastases and hormone-refractory PCa, overexpress AMACR [50]. Immunohistochemical studies have shown that expression of AMACR in prostate tissue has a sensitivity of 97% and a specificity of 100% for the detection of PCa. In conjunction with other markers such as the tumor protein p63, which helps to identify basal cells that are absent in prostate cancer, measuring the expression level of AMACR also can be used for the detection of prostate cancer [51].

Detection at an early stage not only improves the outcome but also reduces mortality in PCa. Although the discovery and use of PSA have revolutionized current PCa detection and treatment, it is not enough. Due to this stage, various molecular modifications or genetic alterations have overtaken the current maximum use of this tumor marker. The use of different PSA derivatives, the discovery of molecular derivatives of PSA, new kallikrein markers, PCA3, and gene rearrangements are leading to a significant improvement in the efficiency of PCa management [24, 25].

1.3 Urothelial cancer (UCa)

The urothelium extends from the renal pelvis to the urethra of the prostate. Urothelial carcinomas (UCa) represent the vast majority of cancers arising in the bladder, and approximately 75% of them are noninvasive within the muscular layer. However, despite the treatment options, there is a high rate of recurrence and, in high-grade tumors, progression to muscle-invasive disease (**Figure 2**). The incidence of UCa increases with age. Most of them are diagnosed in patients over 65 years of age, and it is four times higher in men than in women. One of the reasons for this could be tobacco use, which is known to be a risk factor and is most common in men, although other factors such as the androgen receptor could also play a role [52, 53].

UCa can present a noninvasive phenotype, in which the malignant cells are confined to the urothelial layer, and an invasive phenotype, in which the tumor cells can

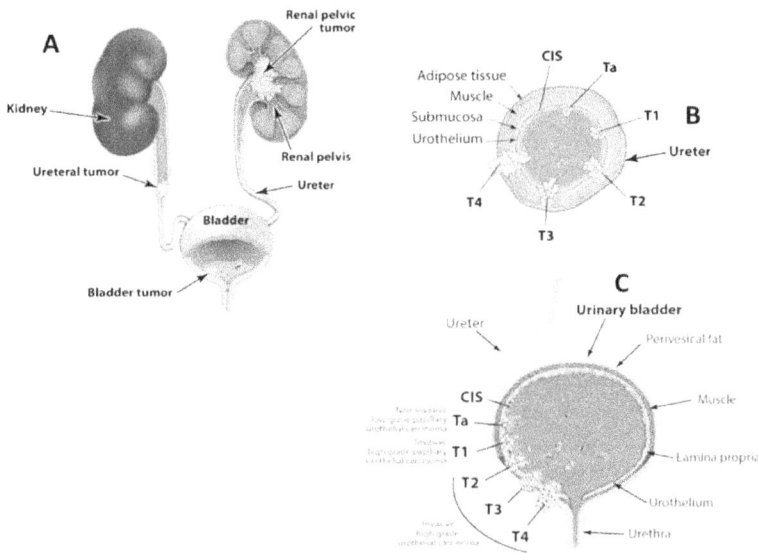

Figure 2.
UCa localization.

break through the basement membrane and invade the subepithelial connective tissue and underlying muscle. There are two types of noninvasive UCa. Exophytic papillary (Ta) tumors are prone to local recurrence but rarely break through the basement membrane or spread. CIS, on the other hand, is a flat lesion with a high susceptibility to invasion and metastasis. Patients who have only CIS lesions in their urinary system are more likely to develop synchronous and/or metachronous malignancies [54]. Ta tumors are caused by molecular abnormalities that are usually separate from CIS and invasive carcinomas, despite the fact that these pathways are not mutually exclusive [55]. The receptor tyrosine kinase-Ras pathway is frequently constitutively active in low-grade papillary carcinomas, with activating mutations in HRAS and FGFR3 [56]. Homozygous deletion of p16INK4a is a common feature in high-grade Ta tumors [57]. TP53 and retinoblastoma (RB) genes and pathways are commonly altered in CIS and invasive malignancies [58]. Although chromosomal-9 deletions can be observed in both dysplastic urothelium and CIS lesions, loss of chromosome 9q heterozygosity is more common in low-grade Ta tumors [59]. When a papillary tumor develops into an invasive phenotype, it is mainly due to the accumulation of additional mutations in the p53 pathway. Invasive cancers have also been shown to have p16 mutations. Matrix metalloproteinases (MMPs), cadherins, TSP-1 (thrombospondin-1), and vascular endothelial growth factors (VEGFs), mutations that alter the extracellular matrix and induce tumor angiogenesis are more common in muscle-invasive cancers and also play a role in nodal metastasis [60].

The most intensively studied aspects of UCa are changes in signaling pathways that affect cell cycle progression. The p53 and Rb signaling pathways, which interact with apoptosis and intracellular signaling mediators, are primarily responsible for cell cycle control. The tumor suppressor gene TP53 is located on chromosome 17p13.1 and encodes the p53 protein. By activating p21WAF1/CIP1, the protein blocks cell cycle progression at the G1-S transition. Inactivation of TP53 and loss of its tumor-suppressive activity may be caused by mutations in the 17p allele [61, 62]. In invasive UCa, loss of heterozygosity on chromosome 17 is associated with aggressive behavior. Mutations in the TP53 gene result in a protein that is resistant to ubiquitin-mediated degradation. Immunohistochemistry can detect increased intranuclear p53 accumulation as a consequence [63]. Multiple retrospective studies have found that accumulation of p53 in the nucleus is associated with poor prognosis in patients with UCa, particularly in those who have undergone radical cystectomy. From normal urothelium to superficial UCa, muscle-invasive cancer and metastatic lymph nodes, altered p53 expression has been observed to occur [64, 65]. Despite this evidence, the predictive function of p53 in the development and progression of bladder cancer is still debated, but what is certain is that a link between the accumulation of p53 in the nucleus and TP53 mutations has been demonstrated [66].

Mdm2 interacts with p53 in an autoregulatory feedback loop that regulates its activity. Increased p53 levels transactivate the promoter of MDM2, causing the translated protein to facilitate the destruction of p53 by the proteasome. MDM2 levels decrease when p53 levels decrease. In UCa, MDM2 amplification has been found to increase in frequency with tumor stage and grade [67, 68]. p14 inhibits the transcription of MDM2. p14ARF, one of two splice variants derived from the CDKN2A locus on chromosome 9p21, encodes the protein. Because the E2F transcription factor induces p14ARF, it serves as a link between the Rb and p53 pathways. The E2F transcription factor is sequestered by dephosphorylated Rb. E2F is produced when Rb is phosphorylated by cyclin-dependent kinases, leading to the transcription of genes important for DNA synthesis [69, 70].

In UCa, a decrease in Rb protein expression has been highlighted. Rb has been shown to be a predictive factor when combined with other cell cycle regulatory proteins. Cyclin/cyclin-dependent kinase complexes help phosphorylate Rb. CDKIs such as p21, p16, and p27, which act as tumor suppressors, cause negative control of cyclin-dependent kinases. Low levels of p27 have been associated with advanced-stage bladder adenocarcinomas [69–71]. In bladder UCa, p27 mutations have also been associated with poor disease-free and overall survival. In UCa patients treated with radical cystectomy, a combined assessment of p53, p21, Rb, cyclin E1, and p27 has been shown to improve accuracy against each individual molecular marker, thereby improving risk stratification [69–71].

Apoptosis is a tightly controlled process involving a series of events that occur during normal development and in response to a series of stimuli, all leading to programmed cell death. Apoptosis can be triggered in two ways. The internal process is mediated by mitochondria, while the extrinsic system involves the activation of death receptors on the cell surface. Both pathways activate caspases that cleave cellular substrates and allow apoptosis. In urothelial carcinoma cell lines, tumor-specific expression of caspase-8 has been shown to induce apoptosis *in vitro* [71].

The Bcl-2 protein family comprises both antiapoptotic and proapoptotic members, such as Bcl-2, Bax, and Bad, and is involved in the intrinsic apoptotic process. In UCa patients treated with radiotherapy or synchronous chemoradiotherapy, increased Bcl-2 expression has been associated with poor outcomes. In patients with advanced UCa undergoing radiotherapy who might benefit from neoadjuvant chemotherapy, Bcl-2 could serve as a marker [72, 73]. Expression of Bcl-2 has been associated with a lower tumor-free survival rate in high-grade T1 tumors, and in combination with p53, it may be a strong prognostic indication in non-muscle-invasive UCa. In addition, a prognostic index based on Mdm2, p53, and Bcl-2 was developed, with abnormalities in all three markers corresponding to the lowest probability of survival in UCa [74, 75]. Bax expression, on the other hand, is an independent predictor of better prognosis in invasive UCa. The proapoptotic function of Bax is mediated by the activation of Apaf-1. In UCa patients, lower Apaf-1 expression has been associated with a higher mortality rate [76, 77].

Multiple cell-surface receptors modify signals from the environment and transmit them to the nucleus of urothelial cells via transduction pathways. Uncontrolled cellular proliferation and tumor growth may result from alterations in these receptors and/ or the signals sent. Activating mutations of FGFR3 are the best-studied alterations in UCa in the FGFR family. FGFR3 mutations are found in nearly 60–70% of low-grade papillary Ta tumors [78].

ErbB-1 and ErbB-2 (Her2/neu), members of the epidermal growth factor receptor (EGFR) family, are overexpressed in invasive UCa. Overexpression of ErbB-1 has been associated with an increased risk of progression and mortality [79]. Increased ErbB-2 expression has also been associated with aggressive UCa as well as poor disease-specific survival. In contrast, other studies have found that ErbB-2 expression is not related to prognosis. While it has been suggested that the combined expression profile of ErbB-1 and ErbB-2 is a stronger predictor of prognosis than either marker alone, this finding remains to be confirmed [80–82].

JAK (Janus kinase) is a tyrosine kinase that is activated by cytokines and growth receptors and regulates a variety of signaling pathways. JAK signaling is thought to be increased by overexpressed preoperative plasma levels of interleukin-6, a ligand for the corresponding cytokine receptor, and is an independent predictor of UCa recurrence and survival [83]. The activation of the STAT (signal transducer and activator of transcription) pathway, which controls transcription of several key genes, is the most studied molecular event after JAK activation. STAT1 inhibits Bcl-2 expression, whereas STAT3 has the reverse effect. In UCa patients, STAT3 expression in combination with other markers can predict the likelihood of recurrence and survival [84].

Angiogenesis is the process of cancer cells producing substances that interact with stromal components to recruit endothelial cells to the site of cancer and generate a vascular supply that gives cancer cells with the nutrients they need to proliferate [85, 86].

VEGFs are signaling proteins that stimulate angiogenesis by interacting with VEGF receptors and stimulating cellular responses (VEGFRs). The majority of known cellular responses to VEGF are mediated by VEGFR2. Advanced UCa and muscle invasion are linked to VEGFR2 expression. In UCa patients, VEGFR2 expression is also a key determinant of nodal metastasis. VEGF boosts nitric oxide synthase, which boosts nitric oxide production and tumor vascularization. In nonmuscle-invasive UCa, VEGF overexpression is linked to early recurrence and progression [87, 88]. VEGFs are signaling molecules that promote angiogenesis by interacting with VEGF receptors and stimulating cellular responses (VEGFRs). The majority of known cellular responses to VEGF are mediated by VEGFR2. Advanced UCa and muscle invasion are linked to VEGFR2 expression. In UCa patients, VEGFR2 expression is also the main predictor of nodal metastasis. VEGF boosts nitric oxide synthase, which boosts nitric oxide production and tumor vascularization. In nonmuscle-invasive UCa, VEGF overexpression is linked to early recurrence and progression [89, 90].

The ability of urothelial cancer cells to invade blood vessels and lymphatics is essential to their ability to spread to nearby structures and form distant metastases. Cadherins are intercellular adhesion mediators that have been identified in a variety of tissues. E-cadherin is the most known member of the cadherin family and is essential for epithelial cell adhesion. In UCa, lower E-cadherin expression has been linked to an increased risk of tumor recurrence and progression and shorter survival [91, 92]. The action of various protease families, including uPAs and MMPs, enhances the ability of a tumor to degrade the matrix and infiltrate the basement membrane. Thymidine phosphorylase (TYMP), an enzyme that increases MMP synthesis, is overexpressed in advanced UCa compared with superficial tumors or normal bladder tissue [93]. Increased thymidine phosphorylase nuclear reactivity has been associated with an increased prevalence of superficial UCa recurrence. MMP-2 and MMP-9 expression levels have been shown to be associated with the stage and grade of urothelial tumors. Increased MMP-2 expression may also indicate a poor prognosis for recurrence-free and disease-specific survival. In UCa patients, the ratio between MMP-9 and E-cadherin is a predictive factor for disease-specific survival [94, 95].

Integrins are transmembrane glycoproteins that can promote tumor development, invasion, and metastasis when their function is disrupted. They are protein receptors for adhesion molecules and collagen. The immunoglobulin superfamily member intercellular adhesion molecule 1 (ICAM1) interacts with particular integrin classes. ICAM1 expression is linked to an infiltrative histological phenotype, according to immunohistochemical investigations. The presence, grade, and size of bladder tumors have all been linked to serum ICAM1 levels [96].

In patients with UCa of the bladder, ICAM1 is part of a multimarker model that can predict nodal status. The α6β4 integrin is tightly connected to collagen VII in normal urothelial cells and inhibits cell migration. Superficial UCa has shown loss of polarity of α6β4 expression, and invasive tumors reveal either loss of α6β4 and/or collagen VII expression or lack of colocalization of either protein. Patients who have malignancies with weak α6β4 immunoreactivity have a better prognosis than those who have tumors with no or significant overexpression. Overall, molecular invasion indicators are relatively accurate predictors of outcome in UCa patients [97].

Circulating tumor cells are the most basic blood-based biomarker. The presence of tumor cells in the blood has been associated with advanced disease stages in various solid organ cancers. In a recent study, the predictive value of the amount of circulating tumor cells obtained with CellSearch technology was investigated in 100 UCa patients who had undergone cystectomy. About 25% of clinically localized Uca patients had circulating tumor cells, the researchers found, and they associated the results with a worse outcome for these patients [98].

Ki-67 is a nuclear protein that is synthesized by proliferating cells that is used to determine the percentage of cell growth fraction. In patients with superficial UCa, the cell proliferative index is associated with prognosis, and the Ki-67 antigen is a strong predictor of progression, recurrence, and treatment response. This result was confirmed in patients receiving cystectomy who had muscle-invasive UCa [99, 100].

Survivin is also an apoptosis inhibitor that can bind caspases after their activation and prevent them from cleaving their substrates. Survivin expression has been shown to be associated with bladder cancer progression and mortality, and its function as a prognostic indicator has been externally validated. In a multiplex panel including other apoptosis-regulating genes, survivin has been shown to predict tumor recurrence after cystectomy and mortality more accurately than clinicopathological factors alone [101].

COX-2 is an enzyme known primarily for being a target for nonsteroidal anti-inflammatory drugs. Increased levels of COX-2 have been studied in both the upper and lower urinary tract as a marker of UCa angiogenesis and tumor aggressiveness. COX-2 was increased not only in upper urinary tract carcinomas but also in nearby nontumor cells (stromal cells), suggesting an association between more aggressive upper urinary tract malignancies and worse prognosis [102, 103].

IGF (insulin growth factor) and IGFBP-3 (insulin growth factor binding protein-3) are circulating proteins that function as growth signal mediators and mitogens, respectively. IGF and IGFBP-3 levels were measured preoperatively in individuals having cystectomy to see if they may be used as blood-based predictors of UCa outcome. Although individual marker levels were not efficient, an association between the two of them (low IGF-adjusted IGFBP-3 levels) was a predictor of distant metastases and poor survival [104].

Periplakin is a protein that is found in normal cellular desmosomes and is encoded by the PPL gene. In a cohort study of UCa patients, serum circulating periplakin was investigated and compared to 30 healthy subjects. While UCa patients had considerably lower serum periplakin levels than controls, this difference was diminished in patients with invasive tumors [105].

Bladder cancer is being more recognized as a disease that cannot be treated merely based on pathologic staging; instead, therapeutic efforts must focus on molecular abnormalities in particular tumors. The formation and course of urothelial malignancies have been better understood, thanks to the availability of advanced molecular profiling and computational methods. Future Uca treatment will rely on consensus marker panels to provide accurate prognosis and therapeutic response predictions in individual patients. The disease will be effectively treated if patients are stratified based on risk factors and tumor expression signatures, followed by optimum surgical treatment and disruption of important signaling pathways through the use of therapies targeting several molecular pathways [106].

1.4 Kidney cancer

Kidney cancer is the fourteenth most prevalent cancer in the world, with men having the ninth most common case and women having the fourteenth most common incidence [107, 108].

Renal cancers in adults include malignant tumors of the renal parenchyma and pelvis, but benign tumors and inflammatory causes should also be considered in the differential diagnosis of a renal mass. The majority of tumors arising from the renal pelvis are urothelial tumors, which account for less than 10% of all renal carcinomas. Renal cell carcinoma (RCC), also known as renal adenocarcinoma, is far more common than benign tumors or other malignancies and accounts for 90% of all kidney cancers. RCC can be divided into several histological subgroups, each with its own clinical features and evolution [109].

The clear cell type of renal cell carcinoma is the most common, accounting for 75% of new cases, followed by the papillary, chromophobe, medullary, and collecting duct subtypes, which account for 10%, 5%, 1%, and 1% of new cases, respectively [107].

Von Hippel and Lindau characterized a vascularized developmental pattern of the retina that was later identified as part of an autosomal dominant disease. Hemangioblastomas, pheochromocytomas, and clear cell renal carcinomas were also common in these patients. Up to 90% of sporadic RCCs have somatic mutations, promoter methylation, or loss of heterozygosity of VHL. The VHL protein is known to function as a substrate recognition component of an E3 ligase and for ubiquitination and degradation of HIF (hypoxia-inducible factors) [110–112].

The alpha subunit of HIF heterodimerizes with HIFβ under hypoxic conditions or in the absence/inactivation of the VHL protein, translocates to the nucleus, and transcribes a variety of genes, including VEGF, PDGF, and TGF. In most spontaneous RCCs, inappropriate activation of this system is a major cause of angiogenesis, invasion, and metastasis [113].

In metastatic or unresectable RCC, targeting the VEGF pathway has been a cornerstone of treatment. In metastatic RCC, small molecule TKI (tyrosine kinase inhibitors) have proven successful in interrupting VEGF signaling, resulting in longer patient survival. Endothelial cells can be stimulated to proliferate and migrate by VEGF and PDGF [113].

The development of an increased blood supply can promote the development of metastatic niches and lead to the spread of the tumor. Because of this significant metastatic potential, no neoadjuvant systemic treatment is currently accepted for RCC with targeted therapies such as sunitinib or pazopanib. These agents are also not approved for adjuvant treatment after nephrectomy. Several studies have failed to demonstrate that adjuvant TKIs or immunotherapies improve survival after definitive surgery, underscoring the need for early intervention with surgery upfront. The most common genetic mutation in RCC is the loss of chromosome 3p. This region contains the PBRM1 gene in addition to VHL (3p21) [114].

PBRM1 is a "gatekeeper" gene that helps in DNA repair, replication, and transcription. Somatic mutations have been detected in 41% of clear cell renal carcinomas, with estimates ranging from 40 to 50%. Loss of PBRM1 is associated with advanced disease stages, a higher grade cancer, and poorer treatment outcomes [115–117].

Mutations on chromosome 3p could indicate an important genetic event, whether inherited or acquired, that drives early carcinogenesis. RCC features a number of genomic changes, including an increase in 5q with TGFB1 and CSF1R, as well as a 14q deletion with the tumor suppressor candidate NRXN3. Loss of 14q has been related to a progression of the disease and a reduced life expectancy [118, 119].

mTOR is a serine/threonine kinase that forms two different complexes with adaptor proteins—mTORC1 and mTORC2. mTORC1 activity was found in more than half of all RCCs. HIF-1α has been demonstrated to promote the expression of REDD1, a proven mTORC1 inhibitor. Stabilization of HIF1 levels under hypoxic environments causes mTOR signaling to be inhibited [120].

Mutations in TSC1 and PTEN may prevent the HIF-1 signaling axis from inhibiting mTOR, resulting in a second, independent mechanism of carcinogenesis. Everolimus as shown in **Figure 3**, suppresses the activity of mTORC1 via binding to FKBP-12 [121, 122].

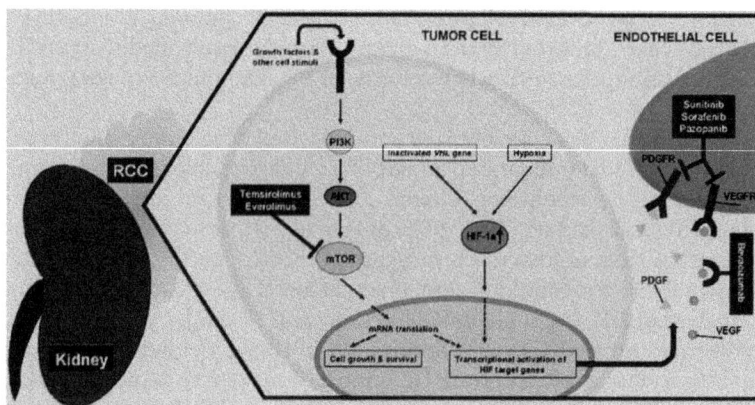

Figure 3.
Current therapeutic management of RCC.

Over the past two decades, research has focused on molecular events that can uncover the biological heterogeneity underlying the diverse clinical behavior of RCC, with the expectation of identifying accurate markers that can personalize prognosis and risk-stratified clinical management, as well as predict response to existing therapeutic approaches [123].

Molecular biomarkers are associated with clinical and/or pathologic characteristics of RCC and have an effect on progression-free survival, OS, cancer-specific mortality, and prognosis [124].

In addition, new research has recently been published on PBRM1 (polybromo 1), BAP1 (BRCA1-associated protein 1), and SETD2 (SET domain-containing protein 2). Although these biomarkers are targeted by a variety of RCC treatments, their prognostic and predictive value has yet to be confirmed internally and externally. All tyrosine kinase inhibitors, such as bevacizumab, target VEGF, while some others, such as cabozantinib, target a larger variety of receptors, including AXL and the protooncogene c-met [123].

As explained earlier, VHL is responsible for the degradation of HIF-α. As a result, changes in VHL proteins lead to HIF-α accumulation in addition to hypoxic cell conditions. HIF-α is a key player in cancer pathogenesis, activating approximately 30 genes involved in tumor proliferation and angiogenesis, including the overexpression of VEGF. When ccRCC (clear cell renal cancer) is compared with papillary or chromophobe forms of RCC, HIF-α expression is significantly higher. In both clear cell and papillary RCC, studies have reported no difference in survival between patients with low or high HIF-α expression, while other studies have found a worse prognosis with increased HIF-α in cancer cells [123].

VEGF is a dimeric glycoprotein that promotes tumor growth and metastasis by influencing angiogenesis in both normal and pathological situations. Due to HIF-α dysregulation and hypoxia caused by an inadequate blood supply in larger tumors, VEGF production is increased in ccRCC. RCC patients with VHL gene mutations and advanced tumor grade have higher VEGF levels and secretion. VEGF expression correlates with tumor necrosis, microvessel invasion, tumor stage, and Fuhrman grade in ccRCC, in addition to tumor grade and size. In studies, increased VEGF levels have been observed to decrease progression-free and overall survival rates of RCC [123, 125].

The additional value of VEGF, despite its promising properties, has yet to be confirmed and externally validated. C-met is a receptor tyrosine kinase and a protooncogene. Angiogenesis, tissue regeneration, cell proliferation, and differentiation are controlled by this protein. Mutations in the c-met signaling pathways have been linked to a variety of tumors, including all forms of RCC [123, 125]. The upregulation of c-met has been linked to the VHL mutation in ccRCC. It has been found that c-met expression is particularly high in tumors with papillary and sarcomatoid differentiation. In recent studies, increased c-met expression was found to reduce cancer-specific mortality. Further research is required to fully understand the role of c-met in the etiology of RCC [126, 127].

Transmembrane protein CAIX is linked to tumor development, poor prognosis, and aggressive phenotype. CAIX is thought to be involved in the regulation of the tumor microenvironment, particularly the fluctuations in intracellular and extracellular pH in response to hypoxia in the tumor, and is regulated by HIF. CAIX is expressed in more than 80% of RCC samples and 90% of ccRCC samples and can therefore be used to confirm the diagnosis of RCC. CAIX expression has been associated with better prognosis and survival in patients with localized RCC and mRCC, and with an inverse relationship with metastatic spread. In contrast, low CAIX expression was not associated with renal cancer mortality [128].

CAIX may be more useful in identifying small renal tumors. With the advancement of technology, three genes have been discovered to be altered in more than 10% of sporadic clear cell RCC: BAP1, PBRM1, and SETD2. We can assume that these genes play an important role in renal cell carcinoma because, as in VHL, they are tumor suppressor genes with two hits found on the short arm of chromosome 3p [129].

The mTOR pathway regulates cell proliferation, protein degradation, and angiogenesis as part of the biological response to environmental stress. PTEN (phosphatase and tensin homolog) is an upstream molecule in this process, while phosphorylated S6 ribosomal protein is a downstream molecule. The use of temsirolimus, an mTOR inhibitor, as a first-line treatment for low-risk patients is recommended in recent treatment guidelines. In addition, recent studies have shown that altering regulators of the mTOR pathway improves the accuracy of prognostic models as well as the ability to predict recurrence in ccRCC patients who had undergone nephrectomy [130, 131].

pS6 (ribosomal protein S6) is a downstream mTOR target that has been associated with the activation of the mTOR pathway. Due to phosphorylated pS6 activity, it exhibits S6 kinase activity that affects mRNA translation. PS6 is overexpressed in clear cell mRCC and could be used to predict survival in both localized and non-localized mRCC. pAkt (protein kinase B) regulates both growth and survival mechanisms by phosphorylating substrates in the cytoplasm and nucleus. Elevated pAkt is associated with lower RCC-specific survival, higher grade, and faster progression of metastasis [123, 132]. Overexpressed pAkt, on the other hand, was linked to a better prognosis in localized RCC. According to recent studies, the localization of pAkt may be essential in defining tumor behavior and thus prognostic value. They discovered a higher level of nuclear pAkt in localized RCC tissue than in mRCC tissue [123, 133].

The tumor suppressor protein PTEN is encoded by the tumor suppressor gene PTEN and is located upstream of mTOR. Via PI3K, PTEN inhibits the phosphorylation of pAkt. PTEN mutation is uncommon in renal cancer and is linked to a high mortality rate. PTEN expression is observed in cancers with a lower T stage and a nonclear cell histological subtype and increases survival [123, 133].

CAF (cytokine and angiogenic factors), survivin, caveolin-1, p53, vimentin, insulin-like growth factor II mRNA-binding protein 3, matrix metalloproteinases, fascin, ki-67, tumor necrosis, and c-reactive protein are examples of other biomarkers. Survivin is a member of the family of apoptosis inhibitors that are active in both the intrinsic and extrinsic caspase pathways [132]. It regulates mitotic progression and promotes alterations in gene expression associated with tumor cell invasiveness. Survivin mRNA is typically expressed during embryonic and fetal development and then disappears in most differentiated adult tissues. Survivin is overexpressed in a variety of malignancies, including all forms of RCC [123].

Given the importance of deregulation of apoptosis in carcinogenesis, it is not surprising that high expression of survivin is associated with poor differentiation, aggressiveness, and lower survival in ccRCC. The p53 protein is a DNA-binding molecule involved in transcription and the regulation of cell growth. When DNA damage occurs, p53 initiates apoptosis and causes cell cycle arrest. Overexpression of p53 has been found in all forms of RCC, especially papillary RCC. Although p53 has been shown to be an independent predictor of metastasis-free survival in patients with localized clear cell RCC, its prognostic significance in RCC is still debated [123].

MMPs are overexpressed in all forms of RCC cancer, especially in nonclear cell RCC tumors, and are associated with aggressive behavior, tumor grade, and survival. Batimastat (synthetic) and bryostatins (natural) are MMP inhibitors that may help to treat and prevent MMP-overexpressing malignancies [123].

IMP3 (insulin-like growth factor II mRNA-binding protein 3) is an RNA-binding protein found in oncofetal tissues. Insulin-like growth factor II mRNA transcription is regulated by it. IMP3 is expressed during embryogenesis in a variety of developing tissues, including epithelium, muscle, and the placenta. In adult tissues, however, it is expressed at low or undetectable levels. In several malignancies, including RCC, IMP3 is associated with cell proliferation and invasion. Stage, grade, sarcomatoid differentiation, regional lymph node involvement, distant metastasis, and cancer-specific mortality are all associated with IMP3. The inclusion of IMP3 expression in the tumor stage increases metastatic progression prediction of metastatic progression and the predictive value of IMP3 in ccRCC was externally validated by researchers [123, 134, 135].

Ki-67 is a cell proliferation marker that has been linked to higher recurrence rates, a more aggressive phenotype of ccRCC, and a poor prognosis. The combination of Ki-67 and CAIX improves the predictive power of nuclear grade in assessing cancer-specific mortality. Complementary studies are needed to evaluate its significance as a prognostic factor [123].

Caveolin-1 is a structural component of caveolae, microdomains of the plasma membrane that regulate cell adhesion, growth, and survival through intracellular signaling. Caveolin-1 is detected in 86% of ccRCCs and 5% of chromophobe and papillary RCCs. The caveolin-1 expression has been linked to a poor clinical outcome in a variety of cancers [123].

One of the components of the scoring algorithm of Leibovich et al. is tumor necrosis. The importance of this component in the prognosis of RCC has led to some debate. When typical clinical and/or pathological tumor features were considered, several studies found that tumor necrosis had no additional value. In contrast, Lam et al. found that tumor necrosis improved survival prediction in patients with localized RCC [136, 137].

The inflammatory marker C-reactive protein has been shown to be a significant predictor of metastasis and overall mortality after nephrectomy for localized renal cell carcinoma. It improved the predictive accuracy of a number of known clinical and pathological predictors by up to 10%. Karakiewicz et al. studied and stated CRP as an independent predictor of mortality in RCC [138].

They also discovered that CRP improved the accuracy of the UISS prediction model. According to Michigan et al., elevated CRP was associated with increased mortality in patients undergoing nephrectomy. Erythrocyte sedimentation rate (ESR), another inflammatory marker, was also associated with higher all-cause mortality. Because they are affordable and readily available, these markers are very promising [123, 127].

Vimentin is a cytoplasmic intermediate filament that should not normally be detected in epithelial cells. Its overexpression has been observed in up to 51% of ccRCC and 61% of papillary RCC, and it has been associated with poor outcomes, regardless of T stage or grade [123].

Fascin is a globular actin cross-link protein that plays a role in cell motility and adhesion. Its overexpression has been associated with sarcomatoid tumors, their stage, grade, size, and metastatic ability [123].

CTLA-4 is a protein described on the surface of cytotoxic T lymphocytes. It is thought to reduce inflammation by preventing tumor-infiltrating lymphocytes (TILs) and T cell activation by preventing tumor cell B71 from binding to CD28. The presence of CTLA-4 has been associated with higher tumor grade in RCC. Lymphocytes also have a cell surface receptor, PD-1. It belongs to the immunoglobulin family and binds to the ligands PD-L1 and PD-L2, which are found on almost all cells, including tumor cells. They are thought to promote apoptosis by decreasing the activity of cytotoxic T cells [139]. In addition, tumor cells are thought to express PD-L1/B7-H1 to prevent tissue destruction by an activated immune system [123, 127].

PD-1 inhibitors, particularly nivolumab, have been the subject of numerous studies, all of which have yielded promising results. The FDA approved nivolumab as second-line therapy for RCC in 2015, based on the results of a study that OS showed benefit, good tolerability, and improved health-related quality of life with nivolumab treatment. It is worth noting that ongoing trials using a mix of targeted treatments, such as anti-VEGFs, and nivolumab are showing promising results [122, 123].

Conflict of interest

The authors declare no conflict of interest.

Author details

Pavel Onofrei[1*], Viorel Dragoş Radu[2*], Alina-Alexandra Onofrei[3], Stoica Laura[1], Doinita Temelie-Olinici[1], Ana-Emanuela Botez[1], Vasile Bogdan Grecu[1] and Elena Carmen Cotrutz[1]

1 Cell and Molecular Biology – Deparment of Morphofunctional Sciences II, "Grigore T. Popa" University of Medicine and Pharmacy, Iasi, Romania

2 Deparment of Surgical Sciences II (Urology), "Grigore T. Popa" University of Medicine and Pharmacy, Iasi, Romania

3 Emergency Hospital for Children "St. Mary", Iasi, Romania

*Address all correspondence to: onofrei.pavel@gmail.com and vioreldradu@yahoo.com

IntechOpen

References

[1] Andre F, Pusztai L. Molecular classification of breast cancer: Implications for selection of adjuvant chemotherapy. Nature Clinical Practice. Oncology. 2006;**3**(11):621-632

[2] Oliveira-Barros EG, Nicolau-Neto P, Da Costa NM, et al. Prostate cancer molecular profiling: The Achilles heel for the implementation of precision medicine. Cell Biology International. 2017;**41**:1239

[3] Gerlinger M, Rowan AJ, Horswell S, et al. Intratumor heterogeneity and branched evolution revealed by multiregion sequencing. The New England Journal of Medicine. 2012; **366**(10):883-892

[4] Karayi MK, Markham AF. Molecular biology of prostate cancer. Prostate Cancer and Prostatic Diseases. 2004; 7(1):6-20

[5] Chial H. Proto-oncogenes to oncogenes to cancer. Nature Education. 2008a;**1**(1):33

[6] Onofrei P, Cotrutz CE, Botez AE, Grecu VB, Solcan C, Sin AI, et al. Maspin and ezrina – Biomarker molecules in colorectal cancer. Correlative immunohistochemical study. Revista de Chimie. 2019;**8**:2926-2933

[7] Olinici D, Cotrutz CE, Mihali CV, Grecu VB, Botez AE, Stoica L, et al. The ultrastructural features of the premalignant oral lesions. Romanian Journal of Morphology and Embryology. 2018;**59**(1):243-248

[8] Olinici D, Solovăstru-Gheucă L, Onofrei P, Cotrutz CE, et al. The molecular mosaic of the premalignant cutaneus lesions. Romanian Journal of Morphology and Embryology. 2016; **57**(2):353-359

[9] Condurache Hritcu OM, Botez AE, Temelie-Olinici D, Onofrei P, Stoica L, Grecu VB, et al. Molecular markers associated with potentially malignant oral lesions (Review). Experimental and Therapeutic Medicine;**22**(2): 834-839

[10] Onofrei P, Olinici D, Sin AI, Stoica L, Botez AE, Grecu VB, et al. A comparative immunohistochemical study regarding the expression of ezrin in colorectal cancer and gastric cancer. Annals of the Romanian Society for Cell Biology. 2017;**21**(3):52-57

[11] LaFleur MW, Muroyama Y, Drake CG, et al. Inhibitors of the PD-1 pathway in tumor therapy. Journal of Immunology. 2018;**200**:375-383

[12] Hanahan D, Weinberg RA. Hallmarks of cancer: The next generation. Cell. 2011;**144**:646-674

[13] Lu P, Weaver VM, Werb Z. The extracellular matrix: a dynamic niche in cancer progression. The Journal of Cell Biology. 2012;**196**:395-406

[14] Kandoth C, Schultz N, Cherniack AD, et al. Integrated genomic characterization of endometrial carcinoma. Nature. 2013;**497**:67-73

[15] Alizadeh AA et al. Towards a novel classification of human malignancies based on gene expression patterns. The Journal of Pathology. 2001;**195**:41-52

[16] Pollack JR. A perspective on DNA microarrays in pathology research and practice. The American Journal of Pathology. 2007;**171**:375-385

[17] Michiels S et al. Prediction of cancer outcome with microarrays: a multiple random validation strategy. Lancet. 2005;**365**:488-492

[18] Ioannidis JP. Microarrays and molecular research: noise discovery? Lancet. 2005;**365**:454-455

[19] Domon B, Aebersold R. Mass spectrometry and protein analysis. Science. 2006;**312**:212-217

[20] Wulfkuhle JD et al. Proteomic approaches to the diagnosis, treatment, and monitoring of cancer. Advances in Experimental Medicine and Biology. 2003;**532**:59-68

[21] Petricoin EF III et al. Serum proteomic patterns for detection of prostate cancer. Journal of the National Cancer Institute. 2002;**94**: 1576-1578

[22] Quackenbush J. Microarray analysis and tumor classification. The New England Journal of Medicine. 2006; **354**:2463-2472

[23] Jemal A, Fedewa SA, Ma J, et al. Prostate cancer incidence and PSA testing patterns in relation to USPSTF screening recommendations. Journal of the American Medical Association. 2015;**314**(19):2054-2061

[24] Jemal A, Fedewa SA, Ma J, et al. Prostate cancer incidence and PSA testing patterns in relation to USPSTF screening recommendations. Journal of the American Medical Association. 2015;**314**(19):2054-2061

[25] Bertsimas D, Silberholz J, Trikalinos T. Optimal healthcare decision making under multiple mathematical models: Application in prostate cancer screening. Health Care Management Science. 2016;**21**(1):105-118

[26] Huang Z, Hurley PJ, Simons BW, et al. Sox9 is required for prostate development and prostate cancer initiation. Oncotarget. 2012;**3**(6): 651-663

[27] Abate-Shen C, Shen MM, Gelmann E. Integrating differentiation and cancer: the Nkx3.1 homeobox gene in prostate organogenesis and carcinogenesis. Differentiation. 2008;**76**(6):717-727

[28] Thomson AA. Mesenchymal mechanisms in prostate organogenesis. Differentiation. 2008;**76**(6):587-598

[29] Donjacour AA, Thomson AA, Cunha GR. FGF-10 plays an essential role in the growth of the fetal prostate. Developmental Biology. 2003;**261**(1): 39-54

[30] Francis JC, Thomsen MK, Taketo MM, et al. Beta-catenin is required for prostate development and cooperates with Pten loss to drive invasive carcinoma. PLoS Genetics. 2013;**9**:e1003180

[31] Mehta V, Schmitz CT, Keil KP, et al. Beta-catenin (CTNNB1) induces Bmp expression in urogenital sinus epithelium and participates in prostatic bud initiation and patterning. Developmental Biology. 2013;**376**:125-135

[32] Simons BW, Hurley PJ, Huang Z, et al. Wnt signaling though beta-catenin is required for prostate lineage specification. Developmental Biology. 2012;**371**:246-255

[33] Catalona WJ, Smith DS, Ratliff TL, et al. Measurement of prostate-specific antigen in serum as a screening test for prostate cancer. The New England Journal of Medicine. 1991;**324**(17): 1156-1161

[34] Partin AW, Carter HB, Chan DW, et al. Prostate specific antigen in the staging of localized prostate cancer: Influence of tumor differentiation, tumor volume and benign hyperplasia. The Journal of Urology. 1990;**143**(4): 747-752

[35] Fair WR, Israeli RS, Heston WD. Prostate-specific membrane antigen. The Prostate. 1997;**32**(2):140-148

[36] Israeli RS, Powell CT, Corr JG, et al. Expression of the prostate-specific membrane antigen. Cancer Research. 1994;**54**(7):1807-1811

[37] Barrett JA, Coleman RE, Goldsmith SJ, et al. First-in-man evaluation of 2 high-affinity PSMA-avid small molecules for imaging prostate cancer. Journal of Nuclear Medicine. 2013;**54**:380-387

[38] Osborne JR, Green DA, Spratt DE, et al. A prospective pilot study of (89) Zr-J591/prostate specific membrane antigen positron emission tomography in men with localized prostate cancer undergoing radical prostatectomy. The Journal of Urology. 2013;**191**:1439-1445

[39] Han S, Woo S, Kim YJ, et al. Impact of 68Ga-PSMA PET on the management of patients with prostate cancer: A systematic review and meta-analysis. European Urology. 2018;**74**:179-190

[40] Becker C, Piironen T, Kiviniemi J, et al. Sensitive and specific immunodetection of human glandular kallikrein 2 in serum. Clinical Chemistry. 2000;**46**:198-206

[41] Lövgren J, Tian S, Lundwall A, et al. Production and activation of recombinant hK2 with propeptide mutations resulting in high expression levels. European Journal of Biochemistry. 1999;**266**:1050-1055

[42] Danila DC, Fleisher M, Scher HI. Circulating tumor cells as biomarkers in prostate cancer. Clinical Cancer Research. 2011;**17**:3903-3912

[43] Yu M, Stott S, Toner M, et al. Circulating tumor cells: approaches to isolation and characterization. The Journal of Cell Biology. 2011;**192**:373-382

[44] Truong M, Yang B, Jarrard DF. Toward the detection of prostate cancer in urine: a critical analysis. The Journal of Urology. 2013;**189**:422-429

[45] de Kok JB, Verhaegh GW, Roelofs RW, et al. DD3(PCA3), a very sensitive and specific marker to detect prostate tumors. Cancer Research. 2002;**62**:2695-2698

[46] Popa I, Fradet Y, Beaudry G, et al. Identification of PCA3 (DD3) in prostatic carcinoma by in situ hybridization. Modern Pathology. 2007;**20**:1121-1127

[47] Hessels D, Klein Gunnewiek JMT, van Oort I, et al. DD3(PCA3)-based molecular urine analysis for the diagnosis of prostate cancer. European Urology. 2003;**44**:8-15

[48] van Gils MPMQ, Hessels D, van Hooij O, et al. The timeresolved fluorescence-based PCA3 test on urinary sediments after digital rectal examination; a Dutch multicenter validation of the diagnostic performance. Clinical Cancer Research. 2007;**13**:939-943

[49] Wozny W, Schroer K, Schwall GP, et al. Differential radioactive quantification of protein abundance ratios between benign and malignant prostate tissues: cancer association of annexin A3. Proteomics. 2007;**7**: 313-322

[50] Luo J, Zha S, Gage WR, et al. Alpha-methylacyl-CoA racemase: A new

molecular marker for prostate cancer. Cancer Research. 2002;**62**:2220-2226

[51] Rubin MA, Zhou M, Dhanasekaran SM, et al. alpha-Methylacyl coenzyme A racemase as a tissue biomarker for prostate cancer. Journal of the American Medical Association. 2002;**287**:1662-1670

[52] Torre LA, Siegel RL, Ward EM, Jemal A. Global cancer incidence and mortality rates and trends--an update. Cancer Epidemiology, Biomarkers & Prevention. 2016;**25**(1):16-27

[53] Antoni S, Ferlay J, Soerjomataram I, Znaor A, Jemal A, Bray F. Bladder cancer incidence and mortality: a global overview and recent trends. European Urology. 2017;**71**(1):96-108

[54] Zehnder P, Moltzahn F, Daneshmand S, Leahy M, Cai J, Miranda G, et al. Outcome in patients with exclusive carcinoma in situ (CIS) after radical cystectomy. BJU International. 2014;**113**(1):65-69

[55] Knowles MA. Molecular subtypes of bladder cancer: Jekyll and Hyde or chalk and cheese? Carcinogenesis. 2006;**27**(3): 361-373

[56] Bakkar AA, Wallerand H, Radvanyi F, Lahaye JB, Pissard S, Lecerf L, et al. FGFR3 and TP53 gene mutations define two distinct pathways in urothelial cell carcinoma of the bladder. Cancer Research. 2003;**63**(23):8108-8112

[57] Orlow I, LaRue H, Osman I, Lacombe L, Moore L, Rabbani F, et al. Deletions of the INK4A gene in superficial bladder tumors. Association with recurrence. The American Journal of Pathology. 1999;**155**(1):105-113

[58] Mitra AP, Datar RH, Cote RJ. Molecular pathways in invasive bladder

cancer: new insights into mechanisms, progression, and target identification. Journal of Clinical Oncology. 2006; **24**(35):5552-5564

[59] Hartmann A, Schlake G, Zaak D, Hungerhuber E, Hofstetter A, Hofstaedter F, et al. Occurrence of chromosome 9 and p53 alterations in multifocal dysplasia and carcinoma in situ of human urinary bladder. Cancer Research. 2002;**62**(3):809-818

[60] Korkolopoulou P, Christodoulou P, Lazaris A, Thomas-Tsagli E, Kapralos P, Papanikolaou A, et al. Prognostic implications of aberrations in p16/pRb pathway in urothelial bladder carcinomas: a multivariate analysis including p53 expression and proliferation markers. European Urology. 2001;**39**(2):167-177

[61] Mitra AP, Hansel DE, Cote RJ. Prognostic value of cell-cycle regulation biomarkers in bladder cancer. Seminars in Oncology. 2012;**39**(5):524-533

[62] Mitra AP, Birkhahn M, Cote RJ. p53 and retinoblastoma pathways in bladder cancer. World Journal of Urology. 2007;**25**(6):563-571

[63] Mitra AP, Lin H, Cote RJ, Datar RH. Biomarker profiling for cancer diagnosis, prognosis and therapeutic management. National Medical Journal of India. 2005;**18**(6):304-312

[64] Chatterjee SJ, Datar R, Youssefzadeh D, George B, Goebell PJ, Stein JP, et al. Combined effects of p53, p21, and pRb expression in the progression of bladder transitional cell carcinoma. Journal of Clinical Oncology. 2004;**22**(6):1007-1013

[65] Shariat SF, Chade DC, Karakiewicz PI, Ashfaq R, Isbarn H, Fradet Y, et al. Combination of multiple

molecular markers can improve prognostication in patients with locally advanced and lymph node positive bladder cancer. The Journal of Urology. 2010;**183**(1):68-75

[66] George B, Datar RH, Wu L, Cai J, Patten N, Beil SJ, et al. p53 gene and protein status: the role of p53 alterations in predicting outcome in patients with bladder cancer. Journal of Clinical Oncology. 2007;**25**(34):5352-5358

[67] Simon R, Struckmann K, Schraml P, Wagner U, Forster T, Moch H, et al. Amplification pattern of 12q13-q15 genes (MDM2, CDK4, GLI) in urinary bladder cancer. Oncogene. 2002;**21**(16):2476-2483

[68] Rebouissou S, Herault A, Letouze E, Neuzillet Y, Laplanche A, Ofualuka K, et al. CDKN2A homozygous deletion is associated with muscle invasion in FGFR3-mutated urothelial bladder carcinoma. The Journal of Pathology. 2012;**227**(3):315-324

[69] Kapur P, Lotan Y, King E, Kabbani W, Mitra AP, Mosbah A, et al. Primary adenocarcinoma of the urinary bladder: Value of cell cycle biomarkers. American Journal of Clinical Pathology. 2011;**135**(6):822-830

[70] Shariat SF, Chromecki TF, Cha EK, Karakiewicz PI, Sun M, Fradet Y, et al. Risk stratification of organ confined bladder cancer after radical cystectomy using cell cycle related biomarkers. The Journal of Urology. 2012;**187**(2):457-462

[71] Karam JA, Lotan Y, Karakiewicz PI, Ashfaq R, Sagalowsky AI, Roehrborn CG, et al. Use of combined apoptosis biomarkers for prediction of bladder cancer recurrence and mortality after radical cystectomy. The Lancet Oncology. 2007;**8**(2):128-136

[72] Ong F, Moonen LM, Gallee MP, ten Bosch C, Zerp SF, Hart AA, et al.

Prognostic factors in transitional cell cancer of the bladder: An emerging role for Bcl-2 and p53. Radiotherapy and Oncology. 2001;**61**(2):169-175

[73] Hussain SA, Ganesan R, Hiller L, Cooke PW, Murray P, Young LS, et al. BCL2 expression predicts survival in patients receiving synchronous chemoradiotherapy in advanced transitional cell carcinoma of the bladder. Oncology Reports. 2003;**10**(3):571-576

[74] Gonzalez-Campora R, Davalos-Casanova G, Beato-Moreno A, Garcia-Escudero A, Pareja Megia MJ, Montironi R, et al. Bcl-2, TP53 and BAX protein expression in superficial urothelial bladder carcinoma. Cancer Letters. 2007;**250**(2):292-299

[75] Maluf FC, Cordon-Cardo C, Verbel DA, Satagopan JM, Boyle MG, Herr H, et al. Assessing interactions between mdm-2, p53, and Bcl-2 as prognostic variables in muscle-invasive bladder cancer treated with neo-adjuvant chemotherapy followed by locoregional surgical treatment. Annals of Oncology. 2006;**17**(11):1677-1686

[76] Korkolopoulou P, Lazaris A, Konstantinidou AE, Kavantzas N, Patsouris E, Christodoulou P, et al. Differential expression of Bcl-2 family proteins in bladder carcinomas. Relationship with apoptotic rate and survival. European Urology. 2002;**41**(3):274-283

[77] Mitra AP, Castelao JE, Hawes D, Tsao-Wei DD, Jiang X, Shi SR, et al. Combination of molecular alterations and smoking intensity predicts bladder cancer outcome: a report from the Los Angeles cancer surveillance program. Cancer. 2013;**119**(4):756-765

[78] van Rhijn BW, Zuiverloon TC, Vis AN, Radvanyi F, van Leenders GJ,

Ooms BC, et al. Molecular grade (FGFR3/MIB-1) and EORTC risk scores are predictive in primary non-muscle-invasive bladder cancer. European Urology. 2010;**58**(3):433-441

[79] Kramer C, Klasmeyer K, Bojar H, Schulz WA, Ackermann R, Grimm MO. Heparin-binding epidermal growth factor-like growth factor isoforms and epidermal growth factor receptor/ErbB1 expression in bladder cancer and their relation to clinical outcome. Cancer. 2007;**109**(10):2016-2024

[80] Kruger S, Weitsch G, Buttner H, Matthiensen A, Bohmer T, Marquardt T, et al. Overexpression of c-erbB-2 oncoprotein in muscle-invasive bladder carcinoma: relationship with gene amplification, clinicopathological parameters and prognostic outcome. International Journal of Oncology. 2002;**21**(5):981-987

[81] Bolenz C, Shariat SF, Karakiewicz PI, Ashfaq R, Ho R, Sagalowsky AI, et al. Human epidermal growth factor receptor 2 expression status provides independent prognostic information in patients with urothelial carcinoma of the urinary bladder. BJU International. 2010;**106**(8): 1216-1222

[82] Kassouf W, Black PC, Tuziak T, Bondaruk J, Lee S, Brown GA, et al. Distinctive expression pattern of ErbB family receptors signifies an aggressive variant of bladder cancer. The Journal of Urology. 2008;**179**(1):353-358

[83] Andrews B, Shariat SF, Kim JH, Wheeler TM, Slawin KM, Lerner SP. Preoperative plasma levels of interleukin-6 and its soluble receptor predict disease recurrence and survival of patients with bladder cancer. The Journal of Urology. 2002;**167**(3): 1475-1481

[84] Mitra AP, Pagliarulo V, Yang D, Waldman FM, Datar RH, Skinner DG, et al. Generation of a concise gene panel for outcome prediction in urinary bladder cancer. Journal of Clinical Oncology. 2009;**27**(24):3929-3937

[85] Bochner BH, Cote RJ, Weidner N, Groshen S, Chen SC, Skinner DG, et al. Angiogenesis in bladder cancer: relationship between microvessel density and tumor prognosis. Journal of the National Cancer Institute. 1995; **87**(21):1603-1612

[86] Bochner BH, Esrig D, Groshen S, Dickinson M, Weidner N, Nichols PW, et al. Relationship of tumor angiogenesis and nuclear p53 accumulation in invasive bladder cancer. Clinical Cancer Research. 1997;**3**(9):1615-1622

[87] Xia G, Kumar SR, Hawes D, Cai J, Hassanieh L, Groshen S, et al. Expression and significance of vascular endothelial growth factor receptor 2 in bladder cancer. The Journal of Urology. 2006;**175**(4):1245-1252

[88] Bernardini S, Fauconnet S, Chabannes E, Henry PC, Adessi G, Bittard H. Serum levels of vascular endothelial growth factor as a prognostic factor in bladder cancer. The Journal of Urology. 2001;**166**(4):1275-1279

[89] Shariat SF, Monoski MA, Andrews B, Wheeler TM, Lerner SP, Slawin KM. Association of plasma urokinase-type plasminogen activator and its receptor with clinical outcome in patients undergoing radical cystectomy for transitional cell carcinoma of the bladder. Urology. 2003;**61**(5):1053-1058

[90] Gazzaniga P, Gandini O, Gradilone A, Silvestri I, Giuliani L, Magnanti M, et al. Detection of basic fibroblast growth factor mRNA in

urinary bladder cancer: Correlation with local relapses. International Journal of Oncology. 1999;**14**(6):1123-1127

[91] Mahnken A, Kausch I, Feller AC, Kruger S. E-cadherin immunoreactivity correlates with recurrence and progression of minimally invasive transitional cell carcinomas of the urinary bladder. Oncology Reports. 2005;**14**(4):1065-1070

[92] Mhawech-Fauceglia P, Fischer G, Beck A, Cheney RT, Herrmann FR. Raf1, aurora-a/STK15 and E-cadherin biomarkers expression in patients with pTa/pT1 urothelial bladder carcinoma; a retrospective TMA study of 246 patients with long-term follow-up. European Journal of Surgical Oncology. 2006;**32**(4):439-444

[93] O'Brien TS, Fox SB, Dickinson AJ, Turley H, Westwood M, Moghaddam A, et al. Expression of the angiogenic factor thymidine phosphorylase/platelet-derived endothelial cell growth factor in primary bladder cancers. Cancer Research. 1996;**56**(20):4799-4804

[94] Aoki S, Yamada Y, Nakamura K, Taki T, Tobiume M, Honda N. Thymidine phosphorylase expression as a prognostic marker for predicting recurrence in primary superficial bladder cancer. Oncology Reports. 2006;**16**(2):279-284

[95] Slaton JW, Millikan R, Inoue K, Karashima T, Czerniak B, Shen Y, et al. Correlation of metastasis related gene expression and relapse-free survival in patients with locally advanced bladder cancer treated with cystectomy and chemotherapy. The Journal of Urology. 2004;**171**(2 Pt 1):570-574

[96] Roche Y, Pasquier D, Rambeaud JJ, Seigneurin D, Duperray A. Fibrinogen mediates bladder cancer cell migration in

an ICAM-1-dependent pathway. Thrombosis and Haemostasis. 2003;**89**(6):1089-1097

[97] Mitra AP, Cote RJ. Molecular signatures that predict nodal metastasis in bladder cancer: Does the primary tumor tell tales? Expert Review of Anticancer Therapy. 2011;**11**(6):849-852

[98] Rink M, Chun FK, Dahlem R, et al. Prognostic role and HER2 expression of circulating tumor cells in peripheral blood of patients prior to radical cystectomy: A prospective study. European Urology. 2012;**61**(4):810-817

[99] Lebret T, Becette V, Herve JM, et al. Prognostic value of MIB-1 antibody labeling index to predict response to bacillus Calmette-Guerin therapy in a high-risk selected population of patients with stage T1 grade G3 bladder cancer. European Urology. 2000;**37**(6):654-659

[100] Margulis V, Lotan Y, Karakiewicz PI, et al. Multi-institutional validation of the predictive value of Ki-67 labeling index in patients with urinary bladder cancer. Journal of the National Cancer Institute. 2009;**101**(2):114-119

[101] Shariat SF, Karakiewicz PI, Godoy G, et al. Survivin as a prognostic marker for urothelial carcinoma of the bladder: A multicenter external validation study. Clinical Cancer Research. 2009;**15**(22):7012-7019

[102] Ke HL, HP T, Lin HH, et al. Cyclooxygenase-2 (COX-2) up-regulation is a prognostic marker for poor clinical outcome of upper tract urothelial cancer. Anticancer Research. 2012;**32**(9):4111-4116

[103] Kang CH, Chiang PH, Huang SC. Correlation of COX-2 expression in stromal cells with high stage, high grade,

and poor prognosis in urothelial carcinoma of upper urinary tracts. Urology. 2008;**72**(1):153-157

[104] Shariat SF, Kim J, Nguyen C, Wheeler TM, Lerner SP, Slawin KM. Correlation of preoperative levels of IGF-I and IGFBP-3 with pathologic parameters and clinical outcome in patients with bladder cancer. Urology. 2003;**61**(2):359-364

[105] Matsumoto K, Ikeda M, Matsumoto T, et al. Serum periplakin as a potential biomarker for urothelial carcinoma of the urinary bladder. Asian Pacific Journal of Cancer Prevention. 2014;**15**(22):9927-9931

[106] Mitra AP, Lerner SP. Potential role for targeted therapy in muscle-invasive bladder cancer: lessons from the cancer genome atlas and beyond. The Urologic Clinics of North America. 2015;**42**(2):201-215

[107] Shuch B, Amin A, Armstrong AJ, et al. Understanding pathologic variants of renal cell carcinoma: Distilling therapeutic opportunities from biologic complexity. European Urology. 2015;**67**:85-97

[108] World Cancer Research Fund. Kidney Cancer Statistics. 2018. Available from: https://www.wcrf.org/dietandcancer/cancer-trends/kidney-cancer-statistics [Accessed date: 09 July 2021]

[109] Chow W, Dong L, Devesa S. Epidemiology and risk factors for kidney cancer. Nature Reviews. Urology. 2010;7(5):245-257

[110] Gossage L, Eisen T. Alterations in VHLas potential biomarkers in renal-cell carcinoma. Nature Reviews. Clinical Oncology. 2010;7(5):277-288

[111] Nordstrom-O'Brien M, van der Luijt RB, van Rooijen E, van den Ouweland AM, Majoor-Krakauer DF, Lolkema MP, et al. Genetic analysis of von Hippel-Lindau disease. Human Mutation. 2010;**31**(5):521-537

[112] Kaelin WG Jr. The von Hippel-Lindau tumour suppressor protein: O2 sensing andcancer. Nature Reviews Cancer. 2008;**8**(11):865-873

[113] Audenet F, Yates DR, Cancel-Tassin G, Cussenot O, Roupret M. Genetic pathways involved in carcinogenesis of clear cell renal cell carcinoma: Genomics towards personalized medicine. BJU International. 2012;**109**(12): 1864-1870

[114] Smaldone MC, Fung C, Uzzo RG, Haas NB. Adjuvant and neoadjuvant therapies in high-risk renal cell carcinoma. Hematology/Oncology Clinics of North America. 2011;**25**(4): 765-791

[115] Duns G, Hofstra RM, Sietzema JG, Hollema H, van Duivenbode I, Kuik A, et al. Targeted exome sequencing in clear cell renal cell carcinoma tumors suggests aberrant chromatin regulation as a crucial step in ccRCC development. Human Mutation. 2012;**33**(7):1059-1062

[116] Varela I, Tarpey P, Raine K, Huang D, Ong CK, Stephens P, et al. Exome sequencing identifies frequent mutation of the SWI/SNF complex gene PBRM1 in renal carcinoma. Nature. 2011;**469**(7331):539-542

[117] Pawlowski R, Muhl SM, Sulser T, Krek W, Moch H, Schraml P. Loss of PBRM1 expression is associated with renal cell carcinoma progression. International Journal of Cancer. 2013;**132**(2):E11-E17

[118] Rydzanicz M, Wrzesinski T, Bluyssen HA, Wesoly J. Genomics and epigenomics of clear cell renal cell carcinoma: Recent developments and potential applications. Cancer Letters. 2013;**341**(2):111-126

[119] Yoshimoto T, Matsuura K, Karnan S, Tagawa H, Nakada C, Tanigawa M, et al. High-resolution analysis of DNA copy number alterations and gene expression in renal clear cell carcinoma. The Journal of Pathology. 2007;**213**(4):392-401

[120] Brugarolas J, Lei K, Hurley RL, Manning BD, Reiling JH, Hafen E, et al. Regulation of mTOR function in response to hypoxia by REDD1 and the TSC1/TSC2 tumor suppressor complex. Genes & Development. 2004;**18**(23): 2893-2904

[121] Kucejova B, Pena-Llopis S, Yamasaki T, Sivanand S, Tran TA, Alexander S, et al. Interplay between pVHL and mTORC1 pathways in clear-cell renal cell carcinoma. Molecular Cancer Research. 2011 Sep;**9**(9): 1255-1265

[122] Motzer RJ, Escudier B, Oudard S, Hutson TE, Porta C, Bracarda S, et al. Efficacy of everolimus in advanced renal cell carcinoma: A double-blind, randomised, placebo-controlled phase III trial. Lancet. 2008;**372**(9637):449-456

[123] Sun M, Shariat SF, Cheng C, Ficarra V, Murai M, Oudard S, et al. Prognostic factors and predictive models in renal cell carcinoma: A contemporary review. European Urology. 2011;**60**(4):644-661

[124] Schmitz-Drager BJ, Droller M, Lokeshwar VB, Lotan Y, Hudson MA, van Rhijn BW, et al. Molecular markers for bladder cancer screening, early diagnosis, and surveillance: the WHO/ICUD consensus. Urologia Internationalis. 2015;**94**(1):1-24

[125] Maroto P, Rini B. Molecular biomarkers in advanced renal cell carcinoma. Clinical Cancer Research. 2014;**20**(8):2060-2071

[126] Gibney GT, Aziz SA, Camp RL, Conrad P, Schwartz BE, Chen CR, et al. c-Met is a prognostic marker and potential therapeutic target in clear cell renal cell carcinoma. Annals of Oncology. 2013;**24**(2):343-349

[127] Ngo TC, Wood CG, Karam JA. Biomarkers of renal cell carcinoma. Urologic Oncology. 2014;**32**(3):243-251

[128] Choueiri TK, Cheng S, Qu AQ, Pastorek J, Atkins MB, Signoretti S. Carbonic anhydrase IX as a potential biomarker of efficacy in metastatic clear-cell renal cell carcinoma patients receiving sorafenib or placebo: analysis from the treatment approaches in renal cancer global evaluation trial (TARGET). Urologic Oncology. 2013;**31**(8):1788-1793

[129] Brugarolas J. PBRM1 and BAP1 as novel targets for renal cell carcinoma. Cancer Journal (Sudbury, Mass). 2013;**19**(4):324-332

[130] Molina AM, Motzer RJ. Clinical practice guidelines for the treatment of metastatic renal cell carcinoma: today and tomorrow. The Oncologist. 2011;**16**(Suppl 2):45-50

[131] Haddad AQ, Kapur P, Singla N, Raman JD, Then MT, Nuhn P, et al. Validation of mammalian target of rapamycin biomarker panel in patients with clear cell renal cell carcinoma. Cancer. 2015;**121**(1):43-50

[132] Li H, Samawi H, Heng DY. The use of prognostic factors in metastatic renal

cell carcinoma. Urologic Oncology. 2015;**33**(12):509-516

[133] Pantuck AJ, Seligson DB, Klatte T, Yu H, Leppert JT, Moore L, et al. Prognostic relevance of the mTOR pathway in renal cell carcinoma: implications for molecular patient selection for targeted therapy. Cancer. 2007;**109**(11):2257-2267

[134] Jiang Z, Chu PG, Woda BA, Liu Q, Balaji KC, Rock KL, et al. Combination of quantitative IMP3 and tumor stage: a new system to predict metastasis for patients with localized renal cell carcinomas. Clinical Cancer Research. 2008;**14**(17):5579-5584

[135] Hoffmann NE, Sheinin Y, Lohse CM, Parker AS, Leibovich BC, Jiang Z, et al. External validation of IMP3 expression as an independent prognostic marker for metastatic progression and death for patients with clear cell renal cell carcinoma. Cancer. 2008;**112**(7): 1471-1479

[136] Leibovich BC, Cheville JC, Lohse CM, Zincke H, Frank I, Kwon ED, et al. A scoring algorithm to predict survivalfor patients with metastatic clear cell renal cell carcinoma: a stratification tool for prospective clinical trials. The Journal of Urology. 2005;**174**(5):1759-1763

[137] Lam JS, Shvarts O, Said JW, Pantuck AJ, Seligson DB, Aldridge ME, et al. Clinicopathologic and molecular correlations of necrosis in the primary tumor of patients with renal cell carcinoma. Cancer. 2005;**103**(12): 2517-2525

[138] Karakiewicz PI, Hutterer GC, Trinh QD, Jeldres C, Perrotte P, Gallina A, et al. C-reactive protein is an informative predictor of renal cell carcinoma-specific mortality: a European study of 313 patients. Cancer. 2007b;**110**(6):1241-1247

[139] Curtis SA, Cohen JV, Kluger HM. Evolving immunotherapy approaches for renal cell carcinoma. Current Oncology Reports. 2016;**18**(9):57

Chapter 3

Control of Cytoskeletal Dynamics in Cancer through a Combination of Cytoskeletal Components

Ban Hussein Alwash, Rawan Asaad Jaber Al-Rubaye,

Mustafa Mohammad Alaaraj and Anwar Yahya Ebrahim

Abstract

The dynamic alterations in the cytoskeletal components actin and intermediate, etc. filaments are required for cell invasion and migration. The actin cytoskeleton is a highly dynamic structure that is governed by a delicate balance of actin filament formation and disassembly. To controlling the activities of key components of the epithelial mesenchymal transition (EMT) could be a viable solution to metastasis. Bioinformatics technologies also allow researchers to investigate the consequences of synthetic mutations or naturally occurring variations of these cytoskeletal proteins. S100A4 is S100 protein family member that interact with a variety of biological target. In study has shown that S100A4 interacts with the tumor suppressor protein p53, indicating that S100A4 may have additional roles in tumor development. The S100A4 and p53 interaction increases after inhibition of MDM2-dependent p53 degradation using Nutlin-3A. The main goal of this research was control of cytoskeletal dynamics in cancer through a combination of, actin and S100A4 protein. The investigate the molecular mechanism behind S100A4 function in (EMT) and indicating that S100A4 is promoting p53 degradation. Understanding the signaling pathways involved would provide a better understanding of the changes that occur during metastasis, which will eventually lead to the identification of proteins that can be targeted for treatment, resulting in lower mortality.

Keywords: cytoskeleton dynamics, actin, cancer, S100A4 protein and p53, bioinformatics

1. Introduction

A highly coordinated multistep process involving the stroma, blood vessels, and cytoskeleton is the leading cause of death in cancer. Invasion, migration, extravasation, and angiogenesis are all important factors in successful metastasis. Invasion is a limited process that occurs at the tumor-host interface, where tumor and stromal cells exchange enzymes and cytokines that modify local ECM and promote cell movement [1]. The ability of cells to move and divide is controlled by dynamic changes. Most cancers are characterized by changes in the expression levels of numerous protein kinases. As a result, most cancer cells show dynamic alterations in cytoskeletal proteins. The capacity of cancer cells to divide, infiltrate, and generate distal metastases is complicated by their migratory nature, the plasticity of cell migration, and these dynamic alterations. The importance of dynamic alterations in the modulation of the function of various cytoskeletal polymers in cancer cells is highlighted in this work. Actin (which generates MF), myosin (mini-filaments), tubulin (MT), and several IF protein families, such as keratins, desmins, peripherin, vimentin, internexins, and others, are among these monomers [2]. The mesenchymal-to-epithelial transition (MET) theory was established to explain these phenomena when histological examinations revealed that macrometastases have epithelial phenotypes rather than mesenchymal phenotypes [3]. DTCs undergo MET to transition from a mesenchymal to an epithelial form, allowing them to multiply at the metastatic site and develop into macrometastases, according to this view. The involvement of the actin cytoskeleton, microtubules, and intermediate filaments in EMT is explored in this paper, as well as how these cytoskeleton proteins can be exploited as a possible biomarker. The S100 family is a subgroup of calcium-binding proteins with EF-hands that regulate a number of cellular processes by interacting with a variety of protein targets. S100A4 expression has been found in fibroblasts, blood cells, and endothelial cells, and it is thought to be one of the mesenchymal cell markers involved in the epithelial-mesenchymal transition (EMT) [4, 5]. The capacity to migrate efficiently in cell motility experiments is a characteristic trait of S100A4-positive cells, but ectopic production of S100A4 in S100A4-negative cells increases migration [6]. Monomers of folded 10S and unfolded extended 6S versions of Nom-muscle myosin (NM IIA) protein exist. The latter has the ability to form filaments [7]. In cancer, genetic changes that impact protein kinases are quite common [8, 9]. Mutations or deletions that induce loss of function or enhanced catalysis are the most common. Activating mutations might have unanticipated consequences for several cytoskeletal systems. Mutations in the small GTPase RhoA, for example, may result in enhanced activation of proteins that regulate minifilament production [10].

These events result in abnormal molecular activities in cancer cells, such as enhanced cell motility, invasion, division, and mechanosensing. The occurrence of many isoforms of these proteins, some of which have non-overlapping activities, complicates the investigation of these alterations. Actin, tubulin, and myosin are all isoforms, and IF comes in a variety of forms and variations. One of the main goals of this project is to present a broad, although incomplete, view of the field. Finding possible areas that could be targeted specifically to treat a variety of cancers in human cancer A431 cells, we show that S100A4 expression is increased during EMT mediated by the transcription factor ZEB2. In addition, we show the interaction between endogenous S100A4 and p53 in cells and that the interaction takes place within the cell nucleus. We also show that knockdown of S100A4 results in stabilization of p53 at the protein level. Further, knockdown of S100A4 is shown to increase the transcriptional activity of p53, resulting in p53-dependent growth arrest [11]. Transgelin (TAGLN) has been shown to have a role in the genesis of proteinuria, although the mechanism by which it does so is unclear. The goal of this research was to look at the involvement of TAGLN in the development of proteinuria. The study's distinctive feature is that it provides an updated, birds-eye view of the global changes in the cytoskeleton, which includes changes in tubulin and intermediate filaments as well as actin and actin binding proteins.

2. The cellular cytoskeleton's role in EMT

The cytoskeleton provides the mechanical strength and integrity that allows cells to maintain their shape and movement. **Figure 1** depicts the situation. As seen in the first step, epithelial cancer cells undergo EMT, losing their cell-cell connections and gaining the potential to penetrate the surrounding tissue parenchyma. These EMT-induced cells can subsequently intravasate into the systemic circulation and survive in the circulation before reaching the target site in the third stage. The cells must then extravasate into the tissue parenchyma in the fourth phase before going into dormancy or becoming micro metastases. MET activation in the fifth phase is required for subsequent improvement and potentially life-threatening mega metastases.

The epithelial cytoskeleton is remodeled during EMT, resulting in cell polarity loss and extracellular matrix remodeling (ECM). The cells then become motile and have the ability to invade [12]. The cytoskeleton's critical function in the EMT process is described in the following sections:

2.1 Cytoskeleton of actin

Actin filament remodeling is linked to EMT [13], and it is one of the most important components of the cytoskeleton. G-actin (globular actin) is a monomeric unit,

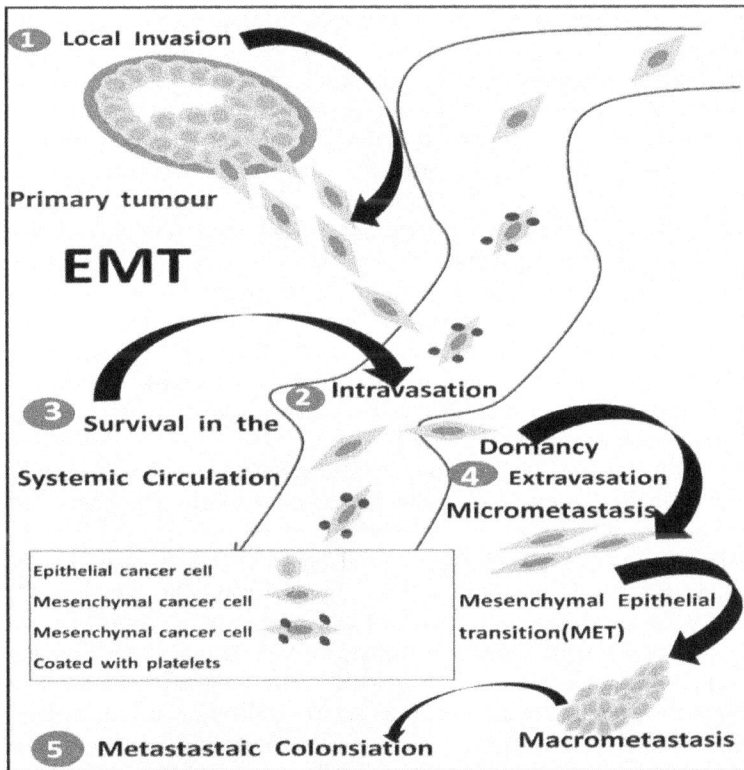

Figure 1.
The metastatic cascade is represented by the EMT-MET model.

while F-actin (fibrous actin) is a polymeric filament. G-actin is distributed uniformly throughout the cytoplasm and nucleus. With the simultaneous hydrolysis of ATP, G-actin rapidly polymerizes to create F-actin under specific physiological conditions. Actomyosin mediates cell spreading and adherence to the ECM by producing conspicuous bundles of F-actin known as stress fibers. Stress fibers attach to focal adhesions and have a function in cell adhesion and morphogenesis as a result. Within the leading cell edge, actin filaments engage with actin-binding proteins and myosin II to deliver F-actin. For cell migration, this is a crucial process. Through its ATP-dependent motor activity, myosin II is thought to play a key role in the construction and disassembly of the actin cytoskeleton [14]. Different biological activities such as cell motility, cell shape, and so on rely on actin organization [15]. Gene expression, post-translational protein modification, and cytoskeleton remodeling all play a role in the EMT process [16]. Recent research has discovered that cells in intermediate phases of EMT have increased tumor-cell spreading ability. E-cadherin complexes have also been demonstrated to be connected to the dynamic actin framework via -catenin and stabilized by inhibiting RhoA activity and activating Rac and cdc42 [13, 17]. Cell-surface receptors, such as integrins, bind to ECM components and play a vital role in altering cell attachment, which is necessary for motility and invasion. A multi-protein complex binds to the actin cytoskeleton and achieves integrin-mediated cell-matrix adhesion.

2.1.1 Proteins that bind to actin

The actin cytoskeleton is made up of actin microfilaments and a large number of actin-binding proteins (ABPs). ABPs are proteins that regulate the formation and disassembly of actin microfilaments. This is important for cell motility, division, and cancer growth, all of which require coordinated actin filament turnover and remodeling [18]. Actin filaments are grouped in a loosely ordered meshwork in lamellipodia, which is referred to as dendritic networks [19], whereas actin filaments are arranged in parallel bundles in filopodia [20]. The action of specific actin-organizing proteins is required for these two types of organizations. During migration, the depolymerization of actin and debranching allows for the dynamic remodeling of the actin network as well as the cyclic extension and retraction of lamellipodia, which generates the pushing force that propels the cell forward. The cell body follows the orientation of the front lamellipodia due to the contraction of actin filaments. Filopodia are made up of closely packed parallel actin filaments with tapered ends facing the plasma membrane. Small crosslinking actin-binding proteins like fascin are principally responsible for bundling filopodia filaments [13, 21].

Cells are thought to be able to penetrate the tissue barrier by forming invadopodia, which are F-actin protrusions that breakdown the ECM, allowing cell penetration [22]. Invadopodia are actin-rich protrusions that are engaged in cell penetration and are related with ECM degradation via local deposition of proteases. The Arp2/3 (actin-related protein2/3) complex is a seven-subunit protein that is regulated by the WAVE and WASP families of WH2 domain-containing proteins (WAVE1, 2, and 3, WASP, and N-WASP), which bind both the Arp2/3 complex and actin monomers [23]. Arp2/3 is a protein complex that aids in the polymerization of actin filaments. Arp2/3 is typically overexpressed in cancers such as breast and liver carcinomas, implying a link between dynamic actin rearrangement and cancer progression [24]. Cortactin, an actin-binding protein, also binds to Arp2/3, allowing active Arp2/3 complexes to be located on the sidewalls of existing actin filaments, resulting in branched arrays of F-actin. Cortactin overexpression has been discovered during metastasis [25, 26].

Facin, an actin-binding protein that stimulates the development of invadopodia and filopodia, is increased during migration [27]. Gelsolin is essential for the formation of lamellipodia and podosomes, both of which are critical protrusions for motile cells [28]. The actin nucleating proteins that regulate cell mobility and organization are known as formins. EMT has been shown to upregulate formin expression at the leading edge in mesenchymal-transformed cells [29]. The gene coding for ABPs has been found to have altered transcription or translation in several cancer types, according to studies. Because ABP expressions vary throughout cancer types, changes in the actin cytoskeleton are a common characteristic of tumor cells. In breast cancer tissues, ARPC2 (actin-related protein2/3 complex) expression is greater and ARPC2 expression is associated with EMT and metastasis [13, 30]. Filamin deficiency has been found to be prevalent in carcinomas such as colon, prostate, and breast cancer [31]. As a result, migration is boosted, which is linked to a bad prognosis [32]. Higher levels of-actinin (actin filament cross-linker) are linked to a bad prognosis in breast cancer, as well as the degree of clinical progression and lymph node status [33].

2.2 Rho GTPases

Rho GTPases play a role in a range of cellular activities, including cell migration, cell polarity, and cell cycle progression, by controlling actin, MT dynamics, and regulating cytoskeleton and cell adhesion dynamics. It has been established that increased expression of Rho GTPases genes associated with a metastatic phenotype in a variety of cancer types, and are tightly related to the actomyosin cytoskeleton's overall control [34]. Rac1, RhoA, and Cdc42 are members of the Rho family of GTPases, which regulate actin cytoskeleton organization such as cytoskeletal dynamics, cell-cell junction assembly/disassembly, and integrin-matrix adhesion. Controlling the activities of Rho GTPases is critical during the growth-factor-induced EMT. Rho signaling activity is controlled by guanine nucleotide exchange factors (GEFs) which catalyze the exchange of GDP to GTP. During growth factor-induced EMT, controlling the activities of Rho GTPases is crucial. Guanine nucleotide exchange factors (GEFs), which catalyze the conversion of GDP to GTP, regulate Rho signaling activity. GTPase-activating proteins (GAPs) facilitate intrinsic GTPase activity to re-form the GDP bound state, which inactivates Rho action. Finally, the inactive GTPase domains and their covalently linked lipid groups engage with the guanine nucleotide dissociation inhibitors (GDIs). As show in **Figure 2**, the GDIs prevent GDP from being dissociated from Rho GTPases, which could inhibit spontaneous activation [35].

Rho GTPase activity in cells is regulated by Rho-dependent factors, as shown in this diagram. GEFs can stimulate Rho-GTPases to engage with downstream actomyosin-regulating effectors by activating the exchange of GDP for GTP, whereas GAPs bind to the GTPase and boost the intrinsic GTPase activity by switching bound GTP to GDP. The GDIs interact with the GDP-bound version of the molecule, preventing GTP binding and thus activation. This illustration is based on Raftopoulou and Hall [36]. Rho GTPases function as molecular switches that cycle between a GDP-bound inactive form and a GTP-bound active form to govern signal transduction pathways [13, 36].

Rho governs cytoskeleton alterations and stimulates actin stress fiber production, impacting cell-cell or cell-matrix adhesion. Rho signaling is important in the regulation of actin-myosin contraction because it stimulates actin reorganization, which leads to the formation of stress fibers. Many of these regulatory mechanisms become unregulated in cancer cells, which contributes to invasive behavior during metastasis, according to recent research [37].

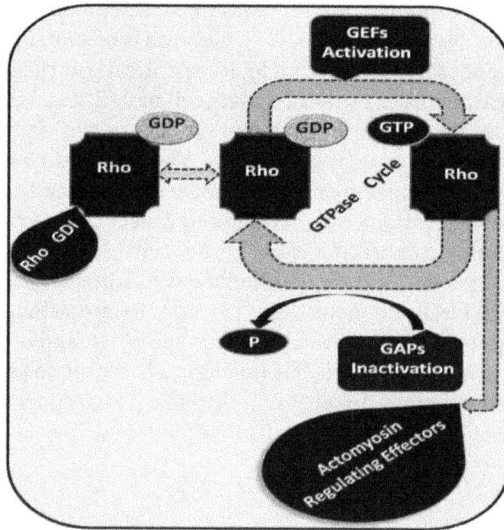

Figure 2.
The diagram depicted Rho GTPase cycle.

2.3 Microtubule (MT)

In EMT, all aspects of the actin cytoskeleton and intermediate filaments are well identified, but the function of microtubules (MT) is still being explored. MTs are an important part of the cytoskeleton and play an important role in movement, intracellular transport and supporting cell shape [38]. MTs are composed of α and β-tubulin dimers, which mostly grow and shrink from the positive end and produce dynamic instability [39]. The function of MTs depends on their assembly and stability, which are regulated by post-translational modifications and interactions with various stable and destabilizing proteins [40]. Calmodulin regulated spectrin associated protein (CAMSAP3) is an MT-binding protein required to maintain MT tissue. It has been shown that the loss of CAMSAP3 promotes Akt dependent EMT through tubulin acetylation [41]. Studies have shown that the microtubule-interacting protein EB1 (end-binding protein) is located in one location and interacts with the microtubules. EB1 is a negative regulator of microtubule stability and promotes the migration of tumor cells. It modulates the dynamics of MT both in vitro and in vivo [42, 43]. Stathmin is an MT regulatory protein that depolymerizes MT and strengthens and regulates MT dynamics. MT destabilization is related to the phosphorylation of stathmin at its four serine residues [44]. In some human cancers, such as Wilms' sarcomas and tumors, stathmin levels have been elevated and have been associated with more aggressive metastases [45]. During EMT, MT plays a significant role in cell migration. Anti-MT drugs act on the one hand by inhibiting cell division, but also by inhibiting cell migration by stopping the formation of projections of MT-based membranes [46, 47]. Stability variability in MT regulates cortical F-actin by activating or inhibiting various Rho GTPases [13, 48]. Aside from their roles in cell division and migration, MT is also important for cell polarization. The creation of a polarized MT required for morphogenesis and cell migration is thought to be aided by cortical control of MT. Although MT indirectly contributes to cell-cell adhesion through dynamic remodeling of the actin network, the role of MT in regulating migration or EMT by interacting with cell-cell adhesion is currently being investigated. Reveal that the MT-interacting protein stathmin is important in cell migration and metastasis via MT-actin cytoskeleton crosstalk [49]. Novel pharmaceutical techniques could be created using this relationship, in which the actin cytoskeleton is targeted via MT, to overcome the toxic effects associated with some actin-based medicines.

2.4 Intermediate filament (IF)

Intermediate filaments (IF) are important cytoskeletal components that provide structural support and mechanical strength. One of the largest gene families in the human genome encodes more than 50 different IF proteins, and this family contains five different IF classes. Types I-IV are located in the cytoplasm and include vimentin, which is a classic marker of EMT, and its expression is related to the aggressive phenotype of epithelial cancer. Compared with actin cytoskeleton and MT, IF also shows a different tissue expression pattern. Type I IF keratin is epithelial-specific and is essential for the mechanical stability of epithelial cells. During EMT, the reduction of keratin is generally considered to be the histological and biochemical characteristics of cancer cells [50, 51]. Type III IF, vimentin, is a typical marker of EMT. Vimentin expression is up-regulated during EMT of epithelial cells, and it has been reported to increase vimentin expression in various cancer cell lines. It is used as an indicator of poor prognosis [52]. During EMT, vimentin helps determine and maintain cell shape. Recent studies have shown that the expression of vimentin is related to active prostate cancer cell lines, and its knockdown significantly reduces the activity and invasiveness of tumor cells [13, 53]. It shows that vimentin is significantly increased in polyploid giant cancer cells (PGCCs). Vimentin intermediate filaments are responsible for expanding morphology and increasing migration [54]. In general, vimentin expression has significant characteristics during EMT, including tumor cell migration and invasion.

3. Materials and methods

The materials and methods are described in the following steps:

3.1 Evaluation of S100A4 and p53 interaction in cells

S100A4 interacts with p53 in the nucleus S100 family proteins have no known enzymatic activity, and therefore it is generally believed that S100 proteins function through interaction with other proteins to regulate their functions. Nuclear colocalization between S100A4 and p53 was however apparent both in untreated and cisplatin-treated A549 cells [11]. Therefore, to investigate the suggested interaction between S100A4 and p53. IP of endogenous S100A4 in A549 cells resulted in coprecipitation of endogenous p53 in untreated cells. In addition, the amount of coprecipitated p53 increased after treatment of the cells with the p53-stabilizing drug Nutlin-3A **Figure 3**. To validate the interaction between S100A4 and p53 and to retrieve information about the subcellular location of the interaction, using antibodies targeting S100A4 and p53 **Figure 3**. The results from PLA supported the interaction between S100A4 and p53 in cells, and also underscored the dramatic increase in the interaction after treatment with Nutlin-3A. In addition, in situ PLA clearly showed that the subcellular location of the interaction between S100A4 and p53 was in the nucleus **Figure 3**.

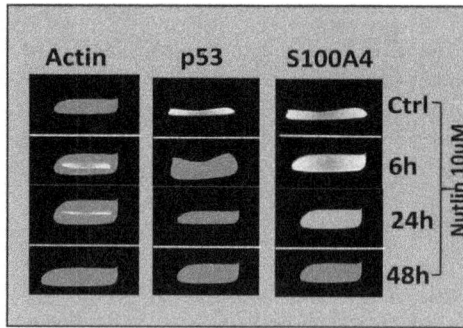

Figure 3.
Immunoblot analysis of p53 and S100A4 protein levels in A549 cells in response to Nutlin-3A treatment at indicated time-points.

3.2 Cytoskeleton protein transgelin developing proteinuria by bioinformatics

The cytoskeleton protein transgelin is designated in the following phases:

3.2.1 Immunity and TAGLN-related transcription factors (TFs) correlation analysis

For stratification of the immune milieu based on function and activity, a group of important immune-related genes that have been widely researched in carcinogenicity were discovered. A scatter plot was used to display statistically significant genes in each category, as well as all relationships within each categorization.

3.2.2 Analysis of the relationship between TAGLN and well-known genes involved in cell viability and apoptosis

According to their function and activity, a group of well-known cancer genes that have been widely examined in carcinogenicity were gathered and divided into cell cycle-related and apoptosis-related pathways. The apoptosis-related star genes were divided into two groups: G0-G1 and G2-M. The expression profile data for each class was used to determine the associations between TAGLN and the star genes.

Differentially expressed genes (DEGs) were identified using Gene Expression Omnibus microarray expression profiling datasets and processed using the short time series expression miner to cluster DEGs in proteinuria progression and build a gene interaction network [55].

3.3 Western blotting

Western blotting dry was used to determine the quantity of extracted P53. In one input, the total protein extracted from cells was displayed, whereas flow-through indicated unbound protein (4-A) [11]. This method was chosen to avoid the presence of antibodies, which could cause more P53 aggregation. To conduct the negative staining experiment, recombinant S100A4 protein was purified under natural conditions. Luciferase IIA immunoprecipitated from A431/ZEB2-WT cells was analyzed using Western blotting [11]. Elution displays the amount of protein that separated from the immunocomplex, while beads reflect the immunocomplex. To see if p53 stabilization alone has an effect on cellular S100A4 levels. Nutlin-3A prevents p53 from interacting with MDM2, the ubiquitin E3 ligase that ubiquitinates p53 and sends it to the proteasome for destruction. We were unable to identify any changes in the messenger RNA (mRNA) level of S100A4, indicating that the increase in S100A4 in response to Nutlin-3A was due to protein stabilization. Knockdown of S100A4 results in increased cisplatin-induced apoptosis S100A4 knockdown by itself did not induce apoptosis, but still the increased p53 levels could prime the cells for apoptosis activation.

3.4 Microscopy with immunofluorescence

Cells were cultured on 9 mm glass coverslips (VWR), fixed with 4% paraformaldehyde (VWR), and permeabilized with 0.5% Triton X-100 (Sigma). Primary and secondary Alexa Fluor conjugated antibodies (Life Technologies) were used for 1 hour of staining. Nuclear staining was done with DAPI (Sigma). An inverted Nikon Eclipse Ti microscope and a custom-built prism-based TIRF microscope with 60× objectives were used for confocal and TIRF microscopy [56]. Samples were analyzed with the help of sample.

4. Result

4.1 In the nucleus S100A4 and p53 interaction

S100A4 interacts with p53 in the nucleus because S100 family members have no known enzymatic activity, it is usually assumed that they control their activities via interacting with other proteins [11]. Non-muscle myosin IIA and p53 have already been identified as possible S100A4-interacting proteins. As a result, we started to look into the possible relationship between S100A4 and p53. In untreated cells, IP of endogenous S100A4 resulted in coprecipitation of endogenous p53.

In addition, as shown in **Figure 4**, the amount of coprecipitated p53 increased after the cells were treated with the p53-stabilizing medication Nutlin-3A. We used

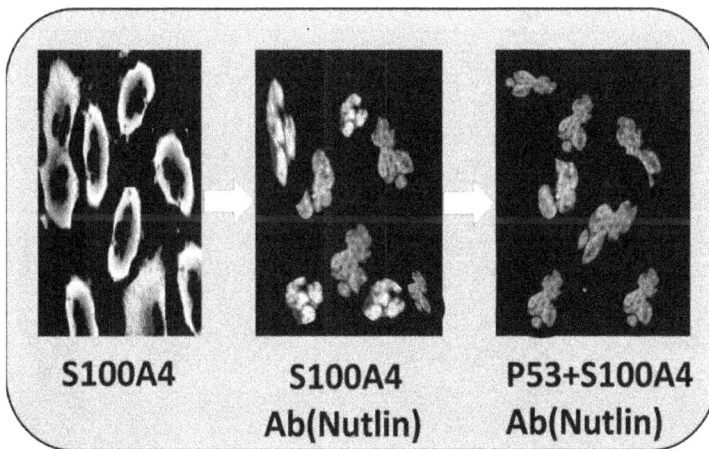

Figure 4.
S100A4 interacts with p53 in the nucleus.

antibodies targeting S100A4 and p53 to perform in situ PLA35 to confirm the interaction between S100A4 and p53 and to acquire information regarding the subcellular location of the interaction. PLA findings confirmed the contact between S100A4 and p53 in cells, as well as the substantial increase in the interaction following Nutlin-3A therapy. Furthermore, in situ PLA clearly demonstrated that the subcellular location of the interaction between S100A4 and p53 was in the nucleus as shown in **Figure 4**.

To utilizing cisplatin, a cytotoxic agent that promotes apoptosis in p53-dependent cells, to see if this was the case. We found higher cisplatin sensitivity in S100A4 shRNA cells relative to control cells using both a short-term cell viability assay and a clonogenic survival experiment as shown in **Figure 5**. We employed different assays to analyze cell mortality after S100A4 knockdown to learn more about the cisplatin response. S100A4 is significantly silenced as shown in **Figure 5**.

4.2 The actin cytoskeleton in EMT: clinical evidence and therapeutic implications

Recent research has revealed that scientists are concentrating their efforts on combination therapies that target numerous molecules in the same signaling pathway, multiple pathways in the same tumor, or both cancer cells and immune cells [57, 58]. Combination medicines are still being studied, and they will help us better understand drug resistance processes in the future. As a result, recent theories propose that targeting EMT and cytoskeletal proteins could be a unique way to battle cancer medication resistance. Normal cell physiology requires actin. As a result, despite their promise in vitro and in vivo, prospective actin-specific chemotherapeutics have yet to be tested. Due to their non-specific targeting of normal tissues, which causes cardiotoxicity and renal difficulties, they have not been successful [59, 60]. Increasing data suggests that the commencement of the EMT process and metastasis causes an increase in the number of EMT-related actin-binding proteins (ABPs) involved with actin cytoskeleton remodeling. As a result, controlling ABP expression may aid in preventing cancer cells from migrating and increasing their sensitivity to

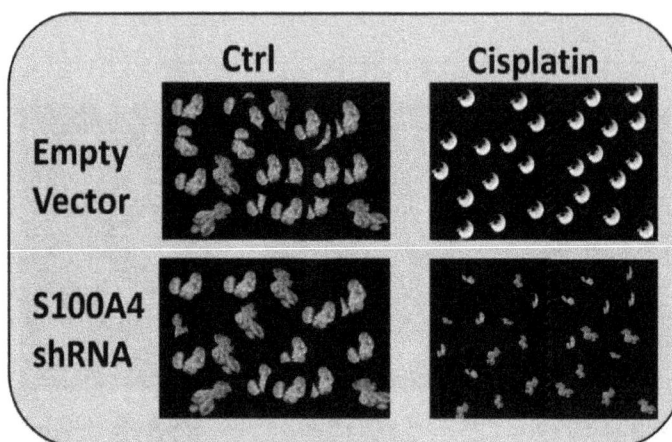

Figure 5.
Knockdown of S100A4 results in increased cisplatin sensitivity.

therapeutic therapies. Arp2/3, cortactin, formins, and fascin have all been studied extensively. Other ABPs, which could be potential targets in carcinogenesis, are, however, understudied. The actin cytoskeleton and ABPs are difficult to target for anti-cancer therapy, because ABPs are involved in the creation of contractile structures in cardiac and skeletal muscles [13, 61]. The intermediate filaments vimentin and nestin are linked to several cancers. When it comes to EMT, vimentin is a marker for mesenchymal cells. Anti-tumor medications have been discovered to change microtubule dynamics, which affect mitosis and apoptosis [62]. Microtubules have a big role in tumor migration and invasion during EMT. These anti-tumor medications stop cancer cells from dividing and forming membrane protrusions caused by network-based microtubules, which cause cell migration and invasion. Eribulin is a MI depolymerization medication that is used to treat metastatic breast cancer patients. In breast cancer, this medication suppresses angiogenesis, vascular remodeling, and EMT [63, 64]. The anti-tumor medication diaryloxazole PC-046 has a high oral bioavailability. It is a synthetically produced small molecule microtubule destabilizing agent. When compared to other microtubule destabilizing agents, this medication is reported to have a lower rate of MDR cross-resistance. Drug resistance in cancer cells is influenced by many signaling pathways involved in EMT and cytoskeletal proteins [65].

Anti-apoptotic effects and drug efflux pumps are increased in EMT cells. As a result, recent theories imply that focusing on EMT and cytoskeletal proteins could be a unique way to battle cancer treatment resistance. Chemotherapy is commonly used in the treatment of cancer, either alone or in combination with radiotherapy or surgery. Multiple breakthroughs in cancer treatment have been made in recent years, while medication resistance, which has been one of the leading causes of cancer death, has increased [66, 67]. In a drug-filled environment, EMT cells are thought to have the ability to develop selectively. While some studies imply that EMT may not totally contribute to cancer metastasis, others reveal that EMT is strongly linked to treatment resistance in cancer cells. Anti-microtubule drug resistance is thought to be caused by changes in the drug target, such as altered microtubule dynamics, tubulin mutations, modified tubulin isotype expression, and altered microtubule regulatory proteins, according to a large body of research. Other cytoskeletal proteins that can regulate microtubule regulation via signaling or structural links have also been discovered may be essential factors of anti-microtubule resistance [68, 69]. ADCs (antibody-drug conjugates) are a new type of targeted anticancer therapy that has been shown to be effective in MDR cancer. When a high-affinity antibody (Ab) binds with the drug and pushes a targeted drug delivery into the cell, this ADC causes apoptosis in tumor cells. In **Figure 6**, aside from producing a cytotoxic load paired with tumor cell death, this Ab-drug combination also blocks the cells' pro-survival receptor. The discovery of ADC could lead to the development of other combination medicines, such as immunotherapy. A lot of work is being done right now to improve the efficacy and targetability of ADCs in the treatment of cancers.

In **Figure 6**, (i) high-affinity antibody binds to the drug. ADC is formed when an antibody binds to a drug and enters the cell's double lipid-membrane layer, causing cell death. (ii) ADC attaches to a cancer cell's pro-survival receptor, blocking its function and triggering apoptosis. (iii) ADC binds to both the cancer cell's membrane-surface antigen and an immune system effector cell, causing cancer cells to be lysed by cellular cytotoxicity.

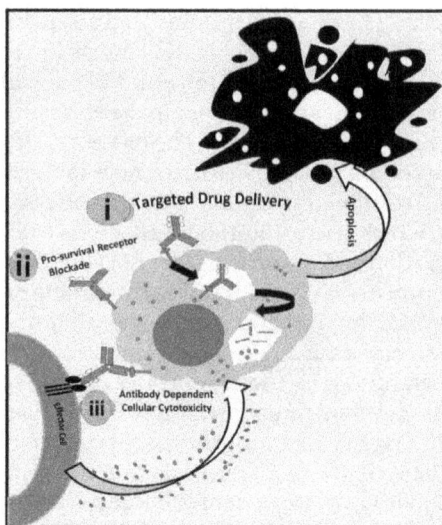

Figure 6.
Diagram depicting the antibody-drug conjugate (ADC) mode of action in a cancer cell.

5. Conclusions

It was necessary to conduct research. The plasticity of the cytoskeleton, motility, multi-drug resistance, and immunosuppressive properties have revealed a great deal about the plasticity of the cytoskeleton, motility, and immunosuppressive properties during the transformation of an epithelial cell to a mesenchymal cell. The cell's signaling systems, and how it adapts in order to live although there has recently been an emphasis on finding new cytoskeletal markers that can be used to detect cancer. Recent research suggests that cytoskeleton dynamics and EMT have a strong association, which can be used to find possible biomarkers. Epithelial cells lose their apical-basolateral polarity and adopt a fibroblast-like motility characteristic during EMT. S100A4 is a mesenchymal marker that is essential for improved mesenchymal cell motility. We chose to study the interactions between NMIIA and S100A4 in a cellular model of EMT because both proteins are expected to work together to generate the mesenchymal cell phenotype. There is less evidence for an S100A4-NMIIA complex in vivo. In this study, we report on control of cytoskeletal dynamics in cancer through a combination of actin and S100A4 protin. The interaction between S100A4 and p53 in the nucleus, and also that S100A4 negatively affects cellular p53 protein levels. In situ PLA was utilized to look at the interaction between p53 and S100A4. We were able to confirm not just the connection between S100A4 and wt p53, but also that it occurs in the cell nucleus, using this method. The difficulties in identifying the connection between p53 and S100A4 might be explained if the interaction between S100A4 and p53 represents a stage in the biological processes that leads to p53 ubiquitination and destruction. Our findings imply that S100A4 is involved in MDM2-dependent p53 ubiquitination and degradation, given the nucleus localization of the interaction between S100A4 and p53 and the fact that lower S100A4 levels result in enhanced p53 stability.

The findings provided here are particularly significant because p53 is one of the most well-known tumor suppressor proteins. An abundance of evidence suggests that p53 inactivation is essentially required for tumor growth. S100A4, a protein that is commonly overexpressed in malignancies and has been linked to poor prognosis, may contribute to p53 degradation through its interaction with p53, according to the findings. These findings clearly indicate why high S100A4 expression is advantageous to tumor development, and they also explain why S100A4 has a poor prognostic impact in clinical trials. Taken together, the findings imply that, in addition to raising the risk of metastasis as previously demonstrated, increased S100A4 expression in malignancies has the ability to suppress p53 activity. This research also suggests that S100A4 expression in clinical samples should be investigated in connection to cisplatin sensitivity to see if S100A4 may be used as a predictor of cisplatin therapy response. Also TAGLN mediated regulatory network implicated in proteinuria development was used. These findings add to our understanding of the molecular pathways driving proteinuria etiology. Recent study has uncovered a significant feature of the protein that makes it a promising candidate for further investigation as a therapeutic target: its specific control of activity levels and expression in cancer cell lines. In both epithelial and mesenchymal cells, the Rho family GTPases play an important role in directing the dynamics of the actin cytoskeleton. There is strong evidence that EMT is linked to the production of the vimentin protein, which is phosphorylated and reoriented in cells, regulating cell contraction and focal adhesion assembly and disassembly. During metastasis, there is also crosstalk between distinct components of the cytoskeleton. The use of actin-binding proteins as new therapeutic targets has a lot of promise for the creation of specific cancer medicines, according to researchers also when employing phenotypic screening to get positive results, there are a lot of procedural concerns to keep in mind. In conclusion, in addition to the crucial role of the RLC phosphorylation in driving the myosin IIA's conformations. These novel findings and analyses are attracting a lot of attention because they have the potential to lead to ground-breaking outcomes in our fight against cancer and drug-resistant cancer cells by combining traditional cancer therapy with EMT-related mechanisms. The findings imply that the mix of cytoskeletal components plays a critical role in the modulation of cytoskeletal dynamics in cancer.

Author details

Ban Hussein Alwash[1], Rawan Asaad Jaber Al-Rubaye[2], Mustafa Mohammad Alaaraj[3] and Anwar Yahya Ebrahim[4*]

1 Faculty of Dentistry, Department of Microbiology, Babylon University, Babylon, Iraq

2 Uclan Medical School, University of Central Lancashire, Uclan, UK

3 Alexandria University, Faculty of Medicine, Alexandria, Egypt

4 University of Babylon, Babylon, Iraq

*Address all correspondence to: anwaralawady@gmail.com

IntechOpen

References

[1] Fares J, Fares MY, Khachfe HH, Salhab HA, Fares Y. Molecular principles of metastasis: A hallmark of cancer revisited. Signal Transduction and Targeted Therapy. 2020;**5**:28

[2] Herrmann H, Bar H, Kreplak L, Strelkov SV, Aebi U. Intermediate filaments: From cell architecture to nanomechanics. Nature Reviews. Molecular Cell Biology. 2007;**8**: 562-573

[3] Banyard J, Bielenberg DR. The role of EMT and MET in cancer dissemination. Connective Tissue Research. 2015;**56**: 403-413

[4] Cabezon T et al. Expression of S100A4 by a variety of cell types present in the tumor microenvironment of human breast cancer. International Journal of Cancer. 2007;**121**:1433-1444

[5] Andersen K et al. The metastasis-promoting protein S100A4 regulates mammary branching morphogenesis. Developmental Biology. 2011;**352**: 181-190

[6] Tarabykina S et al. Metastasis-associated protein S100A4: Spotlight on its role in cell migration. Current Cancer Drug Targets. 2007;7:217-228

[7] Kiboku T, Katoh T, Nakamura A, Kitamura A, Kinjo M, Murakami Y, et al. Nonmuscle myosin II folds into a 10S form via two portions of tail for dynamic subcellular localization. Genes to Cells. 2013;**18**:90-109

[8] Mertins P, Mani DR, Ruggles KV, Gillette MA, Clauser KR, Wang P, et al. Proteogenomics connects somatic mutations to signalling in breast cancer. Nature. 2016;**534**:55-62

[9] Ebrahim AY. Detection of breast cancer in mammograms through a new features technique. In: Tejedor L, Modet SG, Manchev L, Parikesit AA. Breast Cancer and Breast Reconstruction. 2019; IntechOpen. DOI:10.5772/ intechopen.89062. Available from: https://www.intechopen.com/ chapters/69808 [Accessed: 29 October 2019]

[10] Izdebska M, Zielinska W, Grzanka D, Gagat M. The role of actin dynamics and actin-binding proteins expression in epithelial-to-mesenchymal transition and its association with cancer progression and evaluation of possible therapeutic targets. BioMed Research International. 2018;**2018**:4578373

[11] Orre LM et al. S100A4 interacts with p53 in the nucleus and promotes p53 degradation. Oncogene. 2013;**32**(49): 5531-5540

[12] Dongre A, Weinberg RA. New insights into the mechanisms of epithelial-mesenchymal transition and implications for cancer. Nature Reviews. Molecular Cell Biology. 2019;**20**:69-84

[13] Datta A, Deng S, Gopal V, Yap KCH, Halim CE, Lye ML, et al. Cytoskeletal dynamics in epithelial-mesenchymal transition: Insights into therapeutic targets for cancer metastasis. Cancers. 2021;**13**:1882. DOI: 10.3390/ ancers13081882

[14] Anderson TW, Vaughan AN, Cramer LP. Retrograde flow and myosin II activity within the leading cell edge deliver F-actin to the lamella to seed the formation of graded polarity actomyosin II filament bundles in migrating fibroblasts. Molecular Biology of the Cell. 2008;**19**:5006-5018

[15] Grzanka D, Gagat M, Izdebska M. Involvement of the SATB1/F-actin complex in chromatin reorganization during active cell death. International Journal of Molecular Medicine. 2014;**33**:1441-1450

[16] Morris HT, Machesky LM. Actin cytoskeletal control during epithelial to mesenchymal transition: Focus on the pancreas and intestinal tract. British Journal of Cancer. 2015;**112**:613-620

[17] Noren NK, Niessen CM, Gumbiner BM, Burridge K. Cadherin engagement regulates Rho family GTPases. The Journal of Biological Chemistry. 2001;**276**:33305-33308

[18] Ashrafizadeh M, Hushmandi K, Hashemi M, Akbari ME, Kubatka P, Raei M, et al. Role of microRNA/epithelial-to-mesenchymal transition axis in the metastasis of bladder cancer. Biomolecules. 2020;**10**(8):1159

[19] Ashrafizadeh M, Najafi M, Ang HL, Moghadam ER, Mahabady MK, Zabolian A, et al. PTEN, a barrier for proliferation and metastasis of gastric cancer cells: From molecular pathways to targeting and regulation. Biomedicine. 2020;**8**(8):264

[20] Derynck R, Weinberg RA. EMT and cancer: More than meets the eye. Developmental Cell. 2019;**49**:313-316

[21] Hwang ST, Yang MH, Kumar AP, Sethi G, Ahn KS. Corilagin represses epithelial to mesenchymal transition process through modulating Wnt/beta-catenin signaling cascade. Biomolecules. 2020;**10**(10):1406

[22] Shin EM, Hay HS, Lee MH, Goh JN, Tan TZ, Sen YP, et al. DEAD-box helicase DP103 defines metastatic potential of human breast cancers. The Journal of Clinical Investigation. 2014;**124**:3807-3824

[23] Takenawa T, Suetsugu S. The WASP-WAVE protein network: Connecting the membrane to the cytoskeleton. Nature Reviews. Molecular Cell Biology. 2007;**8**:37-48

[24] Sun BO, Fang Y, Li Z, Chen Z, Xiang J. Role of cellular cytoskeleton in epithelial-mesenchymal transition process during cancer progression. Biomedical Reports. 2015;**3**:603-610

[25] Han SP, Gambin Y, Gomez GA, Verma S, Giles N, Michael M, et al. Cortactin scaffolds Arp2/3 and WAVE2 at the epithelial zonula adherens. The Journal of Biological Chemistry. 2014;**289**:7764-7775

[26] Helgeson LA, Prendergast JG, Wagner AR, Rodnick-Smith M, Nolen BJ. Interactions with actin monomers, actin filaments, and Arp2/3 complex define the roles of WASP family proteins and cortactin in coordinately regulating branched actin networks. The Journal of Biological Chemistry. 2014;**289**: 28856-28869

[27] Adams JC. Fascin-1 as a biomarker and prospective therapeutic target in colorectal cancer. Expert Review of Molecular Diagnostics. 2015;**15**:41-48

[28] Chellaiah M, Kizer N, Silva M, Alvarez U, Kwiatkowski D, Hruska KA. Gelsolin deficiency blocks podosome assembly and produces increased bone mass and strength. The Journal of Cell Biology. 2000;**148**:665-678

[29] Jaiswal R, Breitsprecher D, Collins A, Correa IR Jr, Xu MQ, Goode BL. The formin Daam1 and fascin directly collaborate to promote filopodia formation. Current Biology. 2013;**23**:1373-1379

[30] Cheng Z, Wei W, Wu Z, Wang J, Ding X, Sheng Y, et al. ARPC2 promotes

breast cancer proliferation and metastasis. Oncology Reports. 2019;**41**: 3189-3200

[31] Savoy RM, Ghosh PM. The dual role of filamin A in cancer: Can't live with (too much of) it, can't live without it. Endocrine-Related Cancer. 2013;**20**: R341-R356

[32] Zhou H, Zhang Y, Wu L, Xie W, Li L, Yuan Y, et al. Elevated transgelin/TNS1 expression is a potential biomarker in human colorectal cancer. Oncotarget. 2018;**9**:1107-1113

[33] Kovac B, Makela TP, Vallenius T. Increased alpha-actinin-1 destabilizes E-cadherin-based adhesions and associates with poor prognosis in basal-like breast cancer. PLoS One. 2018;**13**:e0196986

[34] Hodge RG, Ridley AJ. Regulating Rho GTPases and their regulators. Nature Reviews Molecular Cell Biology. 2016;**17**(8):496-510

[35] Jaffe AB, Hall A. Rho GTPases: Biochemistry and biology. Annual Review of Cell and Developmental Biology. 2005;**21**:247-269

[36] Raftopoulou M, Hall A. Cell migration: Rho GTPases lead the way. Developmental Biology. 2004;**265**:23-32

[37] Ridley AJ. Rho GTPase signalling in cell migration. Current Opinion in Cell Biology. 2015;**36**:103-112

[38] Olson MF, Sahai E. The actin cytoskeleton in cancer cell motility. Clinical & Experimental Metastasis. 2009;**26**:273-287

[39] Etienne-Manneville S. Microtubules in cell migration. Annual Review of Cell and Developmental Biology. 2013;**29**: 471-499

[40] Toya M, Takeichi M. Organization of non-centrosomal microtubules in epithelial cells. Cell Structure and Function. 2016;**41**:127-135

[41] Luduena RF. A hypothesis on the origin and evolution of tubulin. International Review of Cell and Molecular Biology. 2013;**302**:41-185

[42] Pongrakhananon V, Wattanathamsan O, Takeichi M, Chetprayoon P, Chanvorachote P. Loss of CAMSAP3 promotes EMT via the modification of microtubule-Akt machinery. Journal of Cell Science. 2018;**131**(21):jcs216168

[43] Coquelle FM, Vitre B, Arnal I. Structural basis of EB1 effects on microtubule dynamics. Biochemical Society Transactions. 2009;**37**:997-1001

[44] Zhang T, Zaal KJ, Sheridan J, Mehta A, Gundersen GG, Ralston E. Microtubule plus-end binding protein EB1 is necessary for muscle cell differentiation, elongation and fusion. Journal of Cell Science. 2009;**122**: 1401-1409

[45] Belmont LD, Mitchison TJ. Identification of a protein that interacts with tubulin dimers and increases the catastrophe rate of microtubules. Cell. 1996;**84**:623-631

[46] Baldassarre G, Belletti B, Nicoloso MS, Schiappacassi M, Vecchione A, Spessotto P, et al. p27(Kip1)-stathmin interaction influences sarcoma cell migration and invasion. Cancer Cell. 2005;7:51-63

[47] Landowski TH, Samulitis BK, Dorr RT. The diaryl oxazole PC-046 is a tubulin-binding agent with experimental anti-tumor efficacy in hematologic cancers. Investigational New Drugs. 2013;**31**:1616-1625

[48] Li WT, Yeh TK, Song JS, Yang YN, Chen TW, Lin CH, et al. BPROC305, an orally active microtubule-disrupting anticancer agent. Anti-Cancer Drugs. 2013;**24**:1047-1057

[49] Etienne-Manneville S, Hall A. Integrin-mediated activation of Cdc42 controls cell polarity in migrating astrocytes through PKCzeta. Cell. 2001;**106**:489-498

[50] Byrne FL, Yang L, Phillips PA, Hansford LM, Fletcher JI, Ormandy CJ, et al. RNAi-mediated stathmin suppression reduces lung metastasis in an orthotopic neuroblastoma mouse model. Oncogene. 2014;**33**:882-890

[51] Kim S, Coulombe PA. Intermediate filament scaffolds fulfill mechanical, organizational, and signaling functions in the cytoplasm. Genes & Development. 2007;**21**:1581-1597

[52] Kim S, Kellner J, Lee CH, Coulombe PA. Interaction between the keratin cytoskeleton and eEF1Bgamma affects protein synthesis in epithelial cells. Nature Structural & Molecular Biology. 2007;**14**:982-983

[53] Lang SH, Hyde C, Reid IN, Hitchcock IS, Hart CA, Bryden AA, et al. Enhanced expression of vimentin in motile prostate cell lines and in poorly differentiated and metastatic prostate carcinoma. Prostate. 2002;**52**:253-263

[54] Zhao Y, Yan Q, Long X, Chen X, Wang Y. Vimentin affects the mobility and invasiveness of prostate cancer cells. Cell Biochemistry and Function. 2008;**26**:571-577

[55] Ding Y, Diao Z, Cui H, Yang A, et al. Bioinformatics analysis reveals the roles of cytoskeleton protein transgelin in occurrence and development of

proteinuria. Translational Pediatrics. 2021;**10**(9):2250-2268. DOI: 10.21037/tp-21-83

[56] Badyal SK, Basran J, Bhanji N, Kim JH, Chavda AP, Jung HS, et al. Mechanism of the Ca 2+-dependent interaction between S100A4 and tail fragments of nonmuscle myosin heavy chain IIA. Journal of Molecular Biology. 2011;**405**:1004-1026

[57] Li F, Shanmugam MK, Chen L, Chatterjee S, Basha J, Kumar AP, et al. Garcinol, a polyisoprenylated benzophenone modulates multiple proinflammatory signaling cascades leading to the suppression of growth and survival of head and neck carcinoma. Cancer Prevention Research. 2013;**6**:843-854

[58] Shanmugam MK, Ong TH, Kumar AP, Lun CK, Ho PC, Wong PT, et al. Ursolic acid inhibits the initiation, progression of prostate cancer and prolongs the survival of TRAMP mice by modulating pro-inflammatory pathways. PLoS One. 2012;7:e32476

[59] Newman DJ, Cragg GM. Marine natural products and related compounds in clinical and advanced preclinical trials. Journal of Natural Products. 2004;**67**:1216-1238

[60] Senderowicz AM, Kaur G, Sainz E, Laing C, Inman WD, Rodriguez J, et al. Jasplakinolide's inhibition of the growth of prostate carcinoma cells in vitro with disruption of the actin cytoskeleton. Journal of the National Cancer Institute. 1995;**87**:46-51

[61] Izdebska M, Zielinska W, Halas-Wisniewska M, Grzanka A. Involvement of actin and actin-binding proteins in carcinogenesis. Cell. 2020;**9**(10):2245.9

[62] Manu KA, Shanmugam MK, Li F, Chen L, Siveen KS, Ahn KS, et al. Simvastatin sensitizes human gastric cancer xenograft in nude mice to capecitabine by suppressing nuclear factor-kappa B-regulated gene products. Journal of Molecular Medicine. 2014;**92**: 267-276

[63] Pedersini R, Vassalli L, Claps M, Tulla A, Rodella F, Grisanti S, et al. Eribulin in heavily pretreated metastatic breast cancer patients in the real world: A retrospective study. Oncology. 2018;**94**(Suppl. S1):10-15

[64] Pizzuti L, Krasniqi E, Barchiesi G, Mazzotta M, Barba M, Amodio A, et al. Eribulin in triple negative metastatic breast cancer: Critic interpretation of current evidence and projection for future scenarios. Journal of Cancer. 2019;**10**:5903-5914

[65] Monisha J, Roy NK, Padmavathi G, Banik K, Bordoloi D, Khwairakpam AD, et al. NGAL is downregulated in oral squamous cell carcinoma and leads to increased survival, proliferation, migration and chemoresistance. Cancers. 2018;**10**(7):228

[66] Manu KA, Shanmugam MK, Ramachandran L, Li F, Siveen KS, Chinnathambi A, et al. Isorhamnetin augments the anti-tumor effect of capecitabine through the negative regulation of NF-kappaB signaling cascade in gastric cancer. Cancer Letters. 2015;**363**:28-36

[67] Deng S, Shanmugam MK, Kumar AP, Yap CT, Sethi G, Bishayee A. Targeting autophagy using natural compounds for cancer prevention and therapy. Cancer. 2019;**125**:1228-1246

[68] Mishra S, Verma SS, Rai V, Awasthee N, Chava S, Hui KM, et al.

Long non-coding RNAs are emerging targets of phytochemicals for cancer and other chronic diseases. Cellular and Molecular Life Sciences. 2019;**76**: 1947-1966

[69] Verrills N, Kavallaris M. Improving the targeting of tubulin-binding agents: Lessons from drug resistance studies. Current Pharmaceutical Design. 2005;**11**:1719-1733

Chapter 4

Identification of Biomarkers Associated with Cancer Using Integrated Bioinformatic Analysis

Arpana Parihar, Shivani Malviya and Raju Khan

Abstract

Among the leading cause of death cancer ranked in top position. Early diagnosis of cancer holds promise for reduced mortality rate and speedy recovery. The cancer associated molecules being altered in terms of under/over expression when compared to normal cells and thus could act as biomarkers for therapeutic designing and drug repurposing. The information about the known cancer associated biomarkers can be exploited for targeting of cancer specifically in terms of selective personalized medicine designing. This chapter deals with various types of biomarkers associated with different types of cancer and their identification using integrated bioinformatic analysis. Besides, a brief insight on integrated bioinformatics analysis tools and databases have also been discussed.

Keywords: Cancer, biomarkers, therapy, computational biology, differentially expressed genes

1. Introduction

Cancer is the dreadful disease in which cells divide uncontrollably and, at a later stage, begin attacking neighboring tissues. Hereditary mutations, toxin exposure, radiation exposure, alcohol usage, smoking, and radical lifestyle changes are all known to cause cancer. Early detection of cancer results in good therapy. The traditional diagnostic procedures of X-ray, CT-scan, and tissue biopsy are unable to detect it at an early stage, resulting in a delay in treatment that has resulted in the death of several people globally due to cancer [1, 2]. Substantial advances in cancer biology have resulted in the discovery of various biomolecules that are especially linked to cancer progression and development, and therefore referred to as "biomarkers." Biomarkers are basically alterations which are cellular, biochemical, and molecular changes that can be used to identify or monitor a normal, abnormal, or just a biological process. They are utilized to test and evaluate pathogenic processes, normal biological processes, and the pharmacological response to a treatment intervention objectively. Biomarkers could be classified based on their chemical nature and functionality that can be identified using transcriptomics, metabolomics, genomics and proteomics (**Figure 1**) [3, 4].

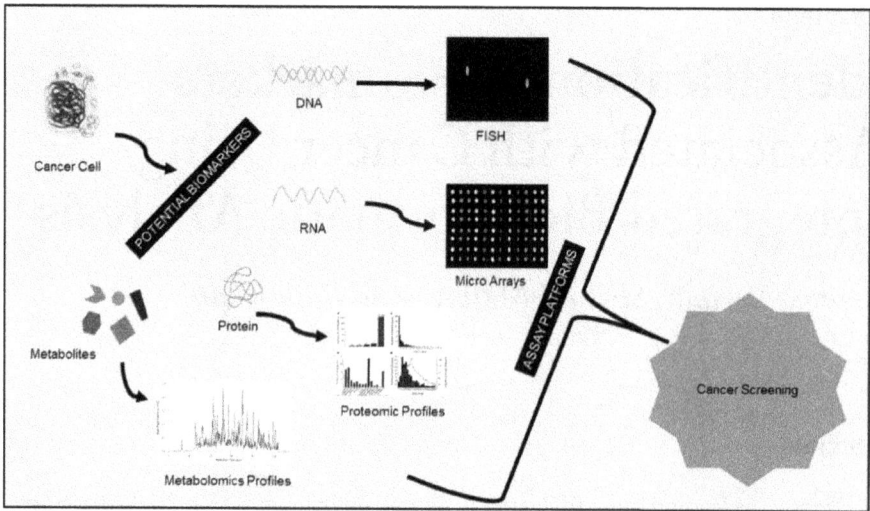

Figure 1.
Analysis of potential biomarkers using different integrated bioinformatics analysis assay platforms such as DNA based from FISH assay platform, RNA based biomarkers from micro arrays, protein based biomarkers from proteomic profiles and metabolites based on biomarkers from metabolomics profiles which led to screening of various kinds of cancer resulting in identification of potential candidate genes for prognostic therapeutic approach.

Usually, living cells have a finite life span, and their genome deoxy ribonucleic acid (DNA) transcribes into ribonucleic acid (RNA), which upon translation results in the creation of proteins that participate in numerous physiological and metabolic processes required by the body. Any change in these mechanisms, such as a mutation in DNA, causes disruption which leads to a dreadful disease namely, Cancer. The detection of mutations in DNA can be used to predict Cancer risk [5]. Consequently, measurement of RNA, protein, and metabolite expression levels can provide important information about illness progression and profiling. There are more than 200 types of cancer reported, however in this chapter, we gathered and presented information about various biomarkers associated with top 5 types of cancer in the world, which can be exploited in designing of sensitive and effective diagnostic technology for early detection of cancer. Basically, various types of biomarkers associated with different types of cancer and their identification using integrated bioinformatic analysis will be discussed. Besides, a brief insight on integrated bioinformatics analysis tools and databases have also been discussed.

2. Biomarkers associated with different types of cancer

Biomarkers have been generally known to play crucial role in the association with different cancer resulting in therapeutic aspects. These could be constructed with the help of advanced integrated bioinformatics analysis tools which could provide an ease to identify biomarkers which could be treated as potential candidates to treat diversities of Cancer. We have listed biomarkers associated with various types of cancer using integrated bioinformatics approaches in **Table 1**. The mechanistic insight regarding how the databases can be utilized to extract and identify various biomarkers associated with respective cancers have been depicted in **Figure 2**.

S. No.	Type of cancer	Biomarkers identified	Investigators	References
1	Lung Cancer	TOP2A, CCNB1, CCNA2, UBE2C, KIF20A, and IL-6	Ni et al., 2018	[6]
2		CDC20, ECT2, KIF20A, MKI67, TPX2, and TYMS	Dai et al., 2020	[7]
3		DDX5, DDX11, DDX55 and DDX56	Cui et al., 2021	[8]
4		NDC80, BUB1B, PLK1, CDC20, and MAD2L1	Liao et al., 2019	[9]
5		UBE2T, UNF2, CDKN3, ANLN, CCNB2, and CKAP2L	Tu et al., 2019	[10]
6		UBE2C, AURKA, CCNA2, CDC20, CCNB1, TOP2A, ASPM, MAD2L1, and KIF11	Liu et al., 2020	[11]
7	Gastric Cancer	CST2, AADAC, SERPINE1, COL8A1, SMPD3, ASPN, ITGBL1, MAP7D2, and PLEKHS1	Liu et al., 2018	[12]
8		FN1, COL1A1, INHBA, and CST1	Wang et al., 2020	[13]
9		COL1A2	Rong et al., 2018	[14]
10		LINC01018, LOC553137, MIR4435-2HG, and TTTY14	Miao et al., 2017	[15]
11		UCA1, HOTTIP, and HMGA1P4	Zang et al., 2019	[16]
12	Liver Cancer	PBK, ASPM, NDC80, AURKA, TPX2, KIF2C, and centromere protein F	Ji et al., 2020	[17]
13		miR1055p, miR7675p, miR12665p, miR47465p, miR500a3p, miR11803p, and miR1395p	Shen et al., 2020	[18]
14		BUB1, CCNB2, CDC20, CDK1, KIF20A, KIF2C, RACGAP1 and CEP55	Li et al., 2017	[19]
15	Breast Cancer	TXN, ANXA2, TPM4, LOXL2, TPRN, ADCY6, TUBA1C, and CMIP	Wang et al., 2019	[20]
16		ADH1A, IGSF10, and the 14 microRNAs	Wu et al., 2021	[21]
17		TPX2, KIF2C, CDCA8, BUB1B, and CCNA2	Cai et al., 2019	[22]
18		CDC45, PLK1, BUB1B, CDC20, AURKA and MAD2L1	Wu et al., 2020	[23]
19	Colorectal Cancer	SLC4A4, NFE2L3, GLDN, PCOLCE2, TIMP1, CCL28, SCGB2A1, AXIN2, and MMP1	Chen et al., 2019	[24]
20		BLACAT1	Dai et al., 2017	[25]
21		HMMR, PAICS, ETFDH, and SCG2	Sun et al., 2021	[26]
22		hsa-miR-183-5p, hsa-miR-21-5p, hsa-miR-195-5p and hsa-miR-497-5p	Falzone et al., 2018	[27]

Table 1.
Biomarkers identified by using integrated bioinformatics tools, associated with various types of cancer such as lung cancer, gastric cancer, colorectal cancer.

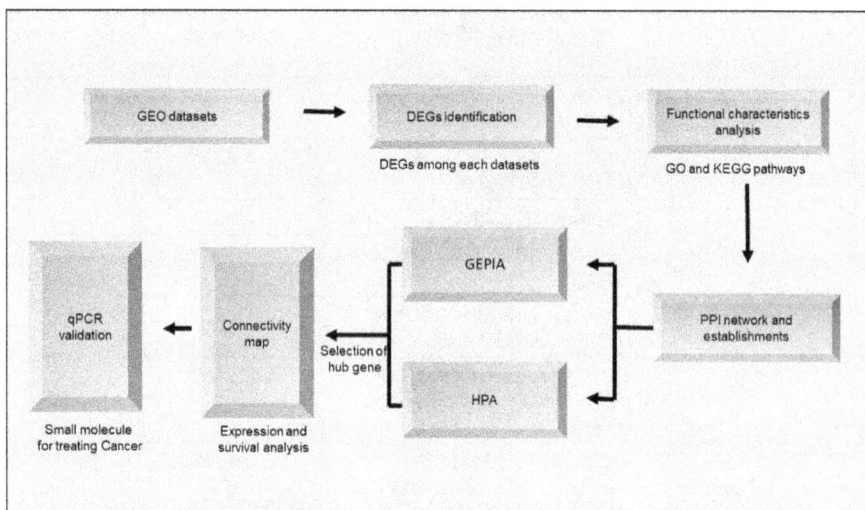

Figure 2.
The schematic representation of extraction of datasets from the GEO database then the identification of DEGs followed by its functional analysis and subsequent qPCR validation leading to identification of small molecule known as biomarker for treating Cancer.

2.1 Lung cancer

Lung cancer is the most common cancer-related death around the globe. Despite great attempts to enhance treatment approaches in previous decades, the clinical outcome of traditional therapies such as surgery, radiation, and chemotherapy remains poor when compared to other major forms of cancer such as colon, prostate, and breast cancers. The challenges in making an early-stage diagnosis of lung cancer and the high recurrence rate after curative treatments are the main reasons for the lack of improvement in prognosis [28]. To improve the clinical result of lung cancer treatments, it is critical to identify and validate diagnostic and prognostic biomarkers. Therefore, here in this section of chapter we have reviewed studies led by certain researchers for identification of the lung cancer biomarkers using integrated bioinformatics analysis. There are mainly 2 types of the lung cancer. In 80–85% cases, the type of lung cancer is non-small cell lung cancer (NSCLC). The main subtypes of which are adenocarcinoma, squamous cell carcinoma, and large cell carcinoma. These subtypes generally begin from different types of the lung cells that are grouped together as NSCLC and their treatment and prognoses are almost similar. The other type is small cell lung cancer (SCLC) and around 10–15% of all lung cancers are SCLC and it is sometimes called oat cell cancer. SCLC grows and spread faster than NSCLC.

In a study by Ni et al., four GEO datasets GSE18842, GSE19804, GSE43458, and GSE62113, were extracted form Gene Expression Omnibus (GEO) database into which the limma package was used to assess differentially expressed genes (DEGs) between NSCLC and normal samples, and the RobustRankAggreg (RRA) programme was used to undertake gene integration. Furthermore, they established the protein–protein interaction (PPI) network of these DEGs using the Search Tool for the Retrieval of Interacting Genes database (STRING), Cytoscape, and Molecular Complex Detection (MCODE). Funrich (http://www.funrich.org) and OmicShare (https://www.omicshare.com/tools/) were also conducted to ensure functional enrichment and pathway enrichment analysis for DEGs. Besides this, they used the gene Expression Profiling Interactive Analysis (GEPIA) and Kaplan Meier-plotter (KM) online datasets to analyze the expressions and prognostic values of top genes. Hence, it led to the identification of a total of 249 DEGs including 113 upregulated and 136 downregulated after gene integration. Followed by this, they established a PPI network with 166 nodes and 1784 protein pairings resulting in TOP2A, CCNB1, CCNA2, UBE2C, KIF20A, and IL-6 to be considered as possible important genes, whereas they further added, the mitotic cell cycle pathway to play a crucial role in NSCLC advancement resulting in its employment as a novel biomarker for NSCLC diagnosis and to guide synthesis medication [6].

In another study by Dai et al., 6 key biomarkers associated with non- small cell lung cancer in which GEO2R were analyzed to examine three microarray datasets from the Gene Expression Omnibus collection along with the enrichment analysis which was performed using Gene Ontology and the Kyoto Encyclopedia of Genes and Genomes. Further, the String database, Cytoscape, and the MCODE plug-in were then used to build a PPI network and screen hub genes using the String database, Cytoscape, and the MCODE plug-in. Kaplan–Meier curves were used to examine overall and disease-free survival of hub genes, as well as the association between target gene expression patterns and tumor grades. To verify enrichment pathways and diagnostic effectiveness of hub genes, researchers performed gene set enrichment analysis and receiver operating characteristic curves. A total of 293 differentially expressed genes were discovered, with cell cycle, ECM–receptor interaction, and malaria being the most prevalent. The PPI network identified 36 hub genes, six of which were reported to have important roles in NSCLC (non- small cell lung cancer) carcinogenesis: CDC20, ECT2, KIF20A, MKI67, TPX2, and TYMS. The target genes discovered can be employed as potential biomarkers to identify and diagnose non- small cell lung cancer as per their investigations [7].

Similarly, in another study by Cui et al., they used integrated bioinformatic analysis of multivariate large-scale databases to assess the potential of DEAD/H box helicases as prognostic indicators and therapeutic targets in lung cancer. They were able to discover four biomarkers with the most significant changes after analyzing the survival and differential expression of these helicases. The unfavorable prognostic factors DDX11, DDX55, and DDX56, as well as the good prognosis factor DDX5, were discovered. MYC signaling is adversely linked with DDX5 gene expression, but favorably associated with DDX11, DDX55, and DDX56 gene expression, according to pathway enrichment analysis led by them. Low mutation levels of TP53 and MUC16, the two most frequently mutated genes in lung cancer, are related with high expression levels of the DDX5 gene. High levels of DDX11, DDX55, and DDX56 gene expression, on the other hand, were linked to high levels of TP53 and MUC16 mutation. The levels of DDX5 gene expression in tumor-infiltrated CD8 + T and B cells are positively correlated, but the other three DEAD box helicases are negatively correlated. Furthermore, while each DDX has a unique miRNA signature, the DDX5-associated miRNA profile is distinct from the miRNA profiles of DDX11, DDX55, and DDX56. The discovery of these four DDX helicases as biomarkers could be considered useful for lung cancer prognostication and targeted treatment development [8].

In another study by Liao et al., they have identified candidate genes associated with the pathogenesis of small cell lung cancer analyzed using integrated bioinformatics tools. GSE60052, GSE43346, GSE15240, and GSE6044 were the four datasets that they downloaded from the Gene Expression Omnibus. R software was used to examine the differentially expressed genes (DEGs) between the SCLC and normal samples. For each dataset, the limma software was utilized. The DEGs from the four datasets were combined using the RobustRankAggreg package. FunRich software and R software were used to conduct functional and route enrichment analyses using the Gene Ontology and Kyoto Encyclopedia of Genes and Genomes databases, accordingly. The DEGs' protein–protein interaction (PPI) network was also built using the STRING database and the Cytoscape software. Molecular Complex Detection in Cytoscape software was used to find hub genes and important modules. Ultimately, the Oncomine online database was used to assess the expression values of hub genes. Following the integration of the four datasets, 412 DEGs were discovered, comprising 146 upregulated genes and 266 downregulated genes. The increased DEGs were mostly involved in cell division, cell cycle, and microtubule binding. The complement and coagulation cascades, the cytokine-mediated signaling pathway, and protein binding were all heavily represented among the downregulated DEGs. Based on a subset of the PPI network, eight hub genes and one major module connected to the cell cycle pathway were discovered. Eventually, in comparison to normal tissue, five hub genes were shown to be substantially expressed in SCLC tissue. The cell cycle route may be the one that is most closely linked to SCLC pathophysiology. As a result, follow-up studies in the diagnosis and therapy of SCLC should focus on NDC80, BUB1B, PLK1, CDC20, and MAD2L1 [9].

In another similar study by Tu et al., GEO2R was used to search the mRNA microarray datasets GSE19188, GSE33532, and GSE44077 for differentially expressed genes (DEGs). The DEGs were analyzed for functional and pathway enrichment using the DAVID database. STRING was used to create a protein–protein interaction (PPI) network, which was then displayed in Cytoscape. MCODE was used to analyze the PPI network's modules. The Kaplan Meier-plotter was used to analyze the overall survival (OS) of genes from MCODE. Total of 221 DEGs were found, with words linked to cell division, cell proliferation, and signal transduction being the most abundant. A PPI network with 221 nodes and 739 edges was created. The PPI network revealed a substantial module containing 27 genes. UBE2T, UNF2, CDKN3, ANLN, CCNB2, and CKAP2L all have high expression levels and have been linked to a poor prognosis in NSCLC patients. Protein binding, ATP binding, cell cycle, and the p53 signaling pathway were among the enriched functions and pathways. DEGs in non- small cell lung cancer (NSCLC) have the potential to be useful targets for diagnosing and treating the disease [10].

In another study by Liu et al., in this prospective investigation, which included 46 tumors and 45 controls, the gene expression profile GSE18842 was acquired from the Gene Expression Omnibus database. They used functional enrichment analysis and KEGG analysis using upregulated differentially expressed genes (uDEGs) and downregulated differentially expressed genes (dDEGs), respectively, after screening differentially expressed genes (DEGs). The STRING database was used to create protein–protein interaction (PPI) networks between DEGs and their corresponding coding protein complexes, which were then examined using Cytoscape. The Kaplan–Meier approach was used to confirm the survival of hub genes. In the TCGA database, the gene expression level heat map of hub genes between NSCLC and neighboring lung tissues was plotted using the GEPIA webserver. After gene integration, they found 368 DEGs (168 uDEGs and 200 dDEGs) in NSCLC samples compared to control samples. They built a PPI network for the DEGs with 249 nodes and 1472 protein pairings on the edges. Survival study confirmed that ten undefined hub genes with the highest connectivity degree (CDK1, UBE2C, AURKA, CCNA2, CDC20, CCNB1, TOP2A, ASPM, MAD2L1, and KIF11) were related with lower overall survival in

NSCLC. The GEPIA web tool was used to verify the expression dependability of hub genes. The findings suggested that UBE2C, AURKA, CCNA2, CDC20, CCNB1, TOP2A, ASPM, MAD2L1, and KIF11 are inherent critical biomarkers for diagnosis and prognosis, and that the mitotic cell cycle pathway is a likely signaling pathway contributing to NSCLC progression, according to KEGG analysis. Such genes could be useful diagnostic biomarkers, as well as a new strategy to designing targeted NSCLC treatments [11].

2.2 Gastric cancer

Despite a substantial drop in incidence and death in North America and most Western European countries in recent decades, gastric cancer (GC) remains the fifth most prevalent malignancy worldwide and poses a serious medical burden, particularly in Eastern Asia [29, 30]. The fact that most patients are discovered at an advanced stage, even with metastatic illnesses, and thus miss out on the potential for a curative resection, accounts for the poor 5-year survival in GC [31, 32]. Substantial progress has been made in comprehending the epidemiology, pathophysiology, and molecular mechanisms of GC, as well as in implementing new therapy alternatives like as targeted and immune-based therapies, not all patients react to molecularly targeted medications developed for specific biomarkers [32, 33]. Hence, due to molecular complexity, poor prognosis, and significant reoccurrence of GC, new diagnostic and prognostic biomarkers are urgently needed [34, 35]. Microarray and high-throughput sequencing technologies have advanced in recent years, allowing researchers to decipher important genetic or epigenetic changes in carcinogenesis and discover promising biomarkers for cancer diagnosis, treatment, and prognosis [36]. Nevertheless, integrated bioinformatics methods have been used in cancer research to overcome limited or inconsistent results due to the use of different technology platforms or a small sample size, and a large range of valuable biological information has been revealed [37–39].

Hence, here we have reviewed a few studies to ensure the role of biomarker identification associated to gastric cancer using integrated bioinformatics analysis tools. In a study by Liu et al., they have considered TOP2A, COL1A1, COL1A2, NDC80, COL3A1, CDKN3, CEP55, TPX2, and TIMP1 which are nine hub genes that may be linked to the etiology of GC. Hence, CST2, AADAC, SERPINE1, COL8A1, SMPD3, ASPN, ITGBL1, MAP7D2, and PLEKHS1 were used to construct a prognostic gene signature that performed well in predicting overall survival. An integrated analysis of several gene expression profile datasets was used by them to find differentially expressed genes between GC and normal gastric tissue samples. Furthermore, protein–protein interaction network and Cox proportional hazards model studies were used to identify key genes related to the pathophysiology and prognosis of GC resulting in their constructed gene signature to be considered as a potential candidate for the biomarker to facilitate the molecular targeting therapy of GC [12].

In a study by Wang et al., they discovered promising biomarkers that could be used to diagnose GC patients. Four Gene Expression Omnibus (GEO) datasets were obtained and examined for differentially expressed genes to look for possible treatment targets for GC (DEGs). The function and pathway enrichment of the discovered DEGs were then investigated using Gene Ontology and Kyoto Encyclopedia of Genes and Genomes (KEGG) analyses. A network of protein–protein interactions (PPI) was created. The degree of connection of proteins in the PPI network was calculated using the CytoHubba plugin of Cytoscape, and the two genes with the highest degree of connectivity were chosen for further investigation. The two DEGs with the highest and lowest log Fold Change values were also chosen. Oncomine and the KaplanMeier plotter platform were used to investigate these six important genes further. A total of 99 genes that were upregulated and 172 genes that were downregulated across all four GEO datasets were examined. The Biological Process phrases 'extracellular matrix organization,' 'collagen catabolic process,' and 'cell adhesion' were primarily enriched in the DEGs. The categories 'ECMreceptor interaction,' 'protein digestion and absorption,' and 'focal adhesion' were considerably enriched in these three KEGG pathways. According to Oncomine, ATP4A and ATP4B expression were downregulated in GC, while all other genes were increased. Upregulated expression of the identified important genes was substantially associated with worse overall survival of GC patients, according to the KaplanMeier plotter platform. The current findings imply that FN1, COL1A1, INHBA, and CST1 could be used as gastric cancer biomarkers and treatment targets. Additional research is needed to determine the role of ATP4A and ATP4B in the treatment of gastric cancer [13].

In another study by Rong et al., their research outlines an integrated bioinformatics approach to identifying molecular biomarkers for stomach cancer in cancer tissues of patients. In large gastric cancer cohorts, they reported distinct expression genes from Gene Expression Ominus (GEO). Their findings found that 433 genes in human stomach cancer have significantly distinct expression patterns. Bioinformatic studies and co-expression network design were used to confirm the different gene expression profiles in gastric cancer. They identified collagen type I alpha 2 (COL1A2), which encodes the pro-alpha2 chain of type I collagen whose triple helix comprises two alpha1 chains and one alpha2 chain, as the key gene in a 37-gene network that modulates cell motility by interacting with the cytoskeleton, based on the co-expression network and top-ranked genes. Immunohistochemistry on human gastric cancer tissue was also used to investigate the predictive function of COL1A2. When compared to normal gastric tissues, COL1A2 was substantially expressed in human gastric cancer. The level of COL1A2 expression was found to be substantially related to histological type and lymph node status after statistical analysis. There were no links found between COL1A2 expression and age, lymph node count, tumor size, or clinical stage. Finally, the unique bioinformatics used in this study led to the discovery of improved diagnostic biomarkers for human stomach cancer, which could aid future research into the crucial change that occurs during the disease's course [14].

In another study, the goal of their research is to find an lncRNA-related signature that can be used to assess the overall survival of 379 GC patients from The Cancer Genome Atlas (TCGA) database. The univariate and multivariate Cox proportional hazards regression models were used to assess the correlations between survival outcome and the expression of lncRNAs. Overall survival was found to be substantially linked with four lncRNAs (LINC01018, LOC553137, MIR4435-2HG, and TTTY14). These four lncRNAs were combined to form a prognostic signature. There was a strong favorable link between overall survival and GC patients with low-risk scores (P = 0.001). Subsequent research found that the predictive usefulness of this four-lncRNA pattern was unaffected by clinical characteristics. These four lncRNAs were linked to many tumor molecular pathways, according to gene set enrichment analysis. Based on bioinformatics analysis, their research suggests that this unique lncRNA expression pattern could be a helpful diagnostic of prognosis for GC patients [15].

The researchers wanted to see if there were any long noncoding RNAs (lncRNAs) that were linked to the pathophysiology and prognosis of GC. The Gene Expression Omnibus (GEO) database was used to retrieve raw noncoding RNA microarray data (GSE53137, GSE70880, and GSE99417). After gene reannotation and batch normalization, an integrated analysis of various gene expression profiles was used to screen for differentially expressed genes between GC and neighboring normal stomach tissue samples. The Cancer Genome Atlas (TCGA) database validated the presence of differentially expressed genes. To identify hub lncRNAs and explore possible biomarkers related to GC diagnosis and prognosis, researchers used a competitive endogenous RNA (ceRNA) network, Gene Ontology term, and Kyoto Encyclopedia of Genes and Genomes pathway, as well as survival analysis. After intersections of differential genes between the GEO and TCGA databases, a total of 246 integrated differential genes were identified, including 15 lncRNAs and 241 messenger RNAs (mRNAs). Three lncRNAs (UCA1, HOTTIP, and HMGA1P4), 26 microRNAs (miRNAs), and 72 mRNAs make up the ceRNA network. Three lncRNAs controlled the cell cycle and cellular senescence, according to functional analyses. The survival rate of HMGA1P4 was statistically connected to the total survival rate, according to a survival analysis. They discovered that HMGA1P4, a miR-301b/miR-508 target, regulates CCNA2 in the GC and is implicated in cell cycle and senescence. Ultimately, three lncRNAs' expression levels were shown to be elevated in GC tissues. As a result, three lncRNAs, UCA1, HOTTIP, and HMGA1P4, may play a role in GC development, and their possible functions may be linked to GC prognosis [16].

2.3 Liver cancer

Liver cancer is among the most frequent malignancies in the world, and it is the second largest cause of cancer death [40, 41]. Due to advances in detection and therapy, people with liver cancer still have a terrible prognosis. Most patients are already in severe stages of symptoms and miss the opportunity to undertake radical resection due to the lack of distinct clinical signs in the early stages. As a result, understanding the pathophysiology of liver cancer aids in early detection, treatment selection, scheduling of follow-up appointments, and prognosis evaluation, all of which can help patients with liver cancer live longer [42]. MicroRNAs (miRNAs) are improperly expressed in a range of tumors and are linked to the pathogenesis of cancers, including liver cancer, according to growing evidence. As tumor suppressor genes or oncogenes, miRNAs play a role in the development of liver cancer. As a result, more research into miRNA expression patterns and consequences could lead to the discovery of new diagnostic or therapeutic targets for liver cancer. Hence, here in this subsection of this chapter we have reviewed certain researches which provide a potential aspect toward identification of biomarkers associated with cancer in relevance to liver utilizing integrated bioinformatics analysis.

Hepatitis B virus (HBV) infection has long been known as a major risk factor for hepatocellular carcinoma (HCC), accounting for at least half of all HCC cases worldwide. Yet, the underlying molecular mechanism of HBV-associated HCC is still unknown. Hence, in an investigation led by Ji et al., they retrieved three microarray datasets from the Gene Expression Omnibus (GEO) collection, including 170 tumoral samples and 181 adjacent normal tissues from the liver of patients with HBV-related HCC which were subjected to integrated analysis of differentially expressed genes (DEGs). Following that, the protein–protein interaction network (PPI) and function and pathway enrichment analyses were carried out. The expression profiles and survival analyses of the ten hub genes selected from the PPI network were carried out. Overall, 329 DEGs were discovered in which 67 were upregulated and 262 were downregulated. PDZ-binding kinase (PBK), abnormal spindle microtubule assembly (ASPM), nuclear division cycle 80 (NDC80), aurora kinase A (AURKA), targeting protein for xenopus kinesin-like protein 2 (TPX2), kinesin family member 2C (KIF2C), and centromere protein F were among the ten DEGs with the highest degree of connectivity (CENPF). Overexpression levels of KIF2C and TPX2 were linked to both poor overall survival and relapse-free survival in a Kaplan–Meier study. Therefore, the hub genes identified in this investigation could be useful in the diagnosis, prognosis, and treatment of HBV-related HCC. Furthermore, their research identifies a number of important biological components (e.g., extracellular exosomes) and signaling pathways that are involved in the progression of HCC caused by HBV, providing a more thorough understanding of the mechanisms underlying HBV-related HCC [17].

In another study by Shen et al., they created nine co-expression modules and discovered that in liver cancer, miR1055p, miR7675p, miR12665p, miR47465p, miR500a3p, miR11803p, and miR1395p were differentially expressed. These miR-NAs were found to have a strong link to the prognosis of patients with liver cancer. MiR1055p and miR1395p may be considered separate prognostic variables among them. As a result, seven miRNAs could be used as predictive indicators in the case of liver cancer [18].

In another study by Li et al., The GSE19665, GSE33006, and GSE41804 microarray datasets were obtained from the Gene Expression Omnibus (GEO) database. Differentially expressed genes (DEGs) were found and function enrichment analyses were carried out. STRING and Cytoscape were used to create the protein–protein interaction network (PPI) and perform module analysis. There were a total of 273 DEGs found, with 189 downregulated genes and 84 upregulated genes. Protein activation, complement activation, carbohydrate binding, complement and coagulation cascades, mitotic cell cycle, and oocyte meiosis are among the DEGs' enhanced activities and pathways. A biological process study found that these genes were primarily abundant in cell division, cell cycle, and nuclear division. BUB1, CDC20, KIF20A, RACGAP1 and CEP55 were found to be involved in the carcinogenesis, invasion, and recurrence of HCC in a survival analysis. Finally, the DEGs and hub genes discovered in this work contribute to our understanding of the molecular pathways underlying HCC carcinogenesis and development, as well as providing candidate targets for HCC diagnosis and treatment [19].

2.4 Breast cancer

Breast cancer is becoming more common over the world, and it is now considered a serious disease among women. Asia has recently emerged as a high-risk location for breast cancer, ranking first among female malignant tumors [43, 44]. Breast cancer therapy has improved recently as a result of constant efforts and advances in contemporary medicine, and the death rate of breast cancer has decreased dramatically. Recurrence and metastasis of breast cancer, on the other hand, have remained unaddressed and have become the most difficult clinical difficulties [43, 45]. To better understand the functions of tumor-related genes and the roles of tumor cell signaling pathways, researchers are turning to genetic studies. Together bioinformatics and system biology are strong multidisciplinary topics that combine biological information collecting, storage, processing, and distribution, summarize life sciences and computer science, and collect and analyze genetic data [46, 47]. Hence, here in this chapter we have reviewed a few studies led by researchers to identify most prevalent biomarkers associated with breast cancer utilizing integrated bioinformatics approaches.

In an investigation by Wang et al. they have analyzed gene expression profiles of GSE48213 using Gene Expression Omnibus database. Further, validation was done using RNA-seq data and clinical information on breast cancer from The Cancer Genome Atlas. In their study, they identified the gene co- expression network which revealed four modules, one of which was found to be strongly linked with patient survival time. They found that the black module which was found to be basal, was made up of 28 genes; the dark red module which was found to be claudin-low, was made up of 18 genes; the brown module which was found to be luminal, was made up of nine genes; and the midnight blue module was made up of seven genes which was investigated to be nonmalignant. Due to a considerable difference in survival time between the two groups, these modules were clustered into two groups. Hence, TXN and ANXA2 in the nonmalignant module, TPM4 and LOXL2 in the luminal module, TPRN and ADCY6 in the claudin-low module, and TUBA1C and CMIP in the basal module were identified by them as the genes with the highest betweenness, implying that they play a central role in information transfer in the network. Therefore, TXN, ANXA2, TPM4, LOXL2, TPRN, ADCY6, TUBA1C, and CMIP are eight hub genes that have been identified and validated by them as being linked to breast cancer progression and poor prognosis to be considered [20].

In another study by Wu et al., Differentially expressed genes (DEGs) in breast cancer were discovered using three data sets from the GEO database. The functional roles of the DEGs were determined using Gene Ontology (GO) enrichment and Kyoto Encyclopedia of Genes and Genomes pathway studies. They also used the Gene Expression Profiling Interactive Analysis (GEPIA), Oncomine, Human Protein Atlas, and Kaplan Meier plotter tool databases to look at the translational and protein expression levels, as well as survival statistics, of DEGs in patients with breast cancer. Using miRWalk and TargetScan, the corresponding change in the expression level of microRNAs in DEGs was predicted, and the expression profiles were evaluated using OncomiR. Finally, RT-qPCR was used to confirm the expression of new DEGs in Chinese breast cancer tissues. ADH1A, IGSF10, and the 14 microRNAs have all been identified as promising new biomarkers for breast cancer diagnosis, therapy, and prognosis [21].

In another study by Cai et al., the Gene Expression Omnibus (GEO) database was used to obtain GSE102484 gene expression profiles. The most potent gene modules related with the metastatic risk of breast cancer were found using weighted gene co-expression network analysis (WGCNA), which yielded a total of 12 modules. 21 network hub genes (MM > 0.90) were kept for further analysis in the most significant module (R2 = 0.68). The biomarkers with the greatest interactions in gene modules were then investigated further using protein–protein interaction (PPI) networks. Five hub genes (TPX2, KIF2C, CDCA8, BUB1B, and CCNA2) were identified as important genes associated with breast cancer progression by the PPI networks. Furthermore, using data from The Cancer Genome Atlas (TCGA) and the Kaplan–Meier (KM) Plotter, the predictive value and differential expression of these genes were confirmed. The mRNA expression levels of these five hub genes have excellent diagnostic value for breast cancer and surrounding tissues, according to a Receiver Operating Characteristic (ROC) curve study. Furthermore, KM Plotter revealed that these five hub genes were substantially related with lower distant metastasis-free survival (DMFS) in the patient group. Five hub genes (TPX2, KIF2C, CDCA8, BUB1B, and CCNA2) linked to the likelihood of distant metastasis were extracted for future study and could be employed as biomarkers to predict breast cancer distant metastasis [22].

In another study by Wu et al., there were a total of 215 DEGs found, with 105 upregulated genes and 110 downregulated genes. The enriched keywords and pathways were primarily linked to cell cycle, proliferation, drug metabolism, and oncogenesis, according to GO and KEGG analyses. Cell Division Cycle 45 (CDC45), Polo Like Kinase 1 (PLK1), BUB1 Mitotic Checkpoint Serine/Threonine Kinase B (BUB1B), Cell Division Cycle 20 (CDC20), Aurora Kinase A (AURKA), and Mitotic Arrest Deficient 2 Like 1 were identified as hub genes from the PPI network (MAD2L1). These hub genes' resilience was confirmed by survival analysis and expression validation tests [23].

2.5 Colorectal cancer

CRC (colorectal cancer) is one of the top causes of death among cancer patients around the world. Older age, male sex, lifestyle, inflammatory bowel illness, and a previous personal history of CRC are all risk factors for the disease. A positive family history is also substantially linked to a higher lifetime relative risk of CRC diagnosis. CRC, on the other hand, is an indolent disease in its early stages, becoming symptomatic only when it evolves to more advanced stages. Numerous attempts have been made to develop adequate screening technologies, but they remain intrusive even now, resulting in reduced attainment rates among large community [48]. Recent breakthroughs in our understanding of the molecular underpinnings and cellular mechanisms of CRC have resulted in the widespread use of particular molecular diagnostics in clinical practice. The patient's risk is stratified and therapy is decided based on the test results. Conversely, current research into biomarkers associated with colorectal cancer could usher in a new age in diagnosis, risk prediction, and treatment selection. Here, we have reviewed a few investigations led to ensure its attainment using integrated bioinformatics analysis [49].

In an investigation led by Chen et al., they analyzed 207 common DEGs in colorectal cancer using the integrated GEO and TCGA databases into which they constructed a PPI network consists of 70 nodes and 170 edges and identified 10 top hub genes. A prognostic gene signature which includes SLC4A4, NFE2L3, GLDN, PCOLCE2, TIMP1, CCL28, SCGB2A1, AXIN2, and MMP1 was constructed by them which revealed overall survival in patients suffering from CRC. Hence, it could be considered as a good potential candidate for further treatments [24].

In a study by Dai et al., they discovered nine differentially expressed lncRNAs and their putative mRNA targets using integrated data mining. They evaluated key pathways and GO words that are associated to the up-regulated and down-regulated transcripts, respectively, after a series of bioinformatics investigations. Meanwhile, qRT-PCR was used to validate the nine lncRNAs in 30 matched tissues and cell lines, and the results were largely compatible with the microarray data. They also looked for nine lncRNAs in the blood of 30 CRC patients with tissue matching, 30 non-cancer patients, and 30 healthy people. Finally, they discovered that BLACAT1 was important for CRC diagnosis. Between CRC patients and healthy controls, the area under the curve (AUC), sensitivity, and specificity were 0.858 (95% CI: 0.765–0.951), 83.3%, and 76.7%, respectively. Furthermore, BLACAT1 exhibited a particular utility in distinguishing CRC from non-cancer disorders. The findings suggest that significantly elevated lncRNAs as well as associated potential target transcripts could be used as therapeutic targets in CRC patients. Conversely, the lncRNA BLACAT1 could be a new supplemental biomarker for CRC detection [25].

In another study by Sun et al., The Gene Expression Omnibus (GEO) mRNA microarray datasets GSE113513, GSE21510, GSE44076, and GSE32323 were collected and processed with bioinformatics to discover hub genes in CRC development. The GEO2R tool was used to look for differentially expressed genes (DEGs). The DAVID database was used to conduct gene ontology (GO) and KEGG studies. To build a protein–protein interaction (PPI) network and identify essential modules and hub genes, researchers employed the STRING database and Cytoscape software. The DEGs' survival studies were done using the GEPIA database. Potential medications were screened using the Connectivity Map database. There were a total of 865 DEGs found, with 374 upregulated and 491 downregulated genes. These DEGs were mostly linked to metabolic pathways, cancer pathways, cell cycle pathways, and so on. With 863 nodes and 5817 edges, the PPI network was discovered. HMMR, PAICS, ETFDH, and SCG2 were found to be strongly linked with overall survival of CRC patients in a survival analysis. Blebbistatin and sulconazole have also been discovered as potential treatments [26].

Falzone et al. used the mirDIP gene target analysis in a sample of 19 differentially expressed miRNAs to determine the interaction between miRNAs and the most changed genes in CRC. DIANA-mirPath prediction analysis was used to identify miRNAs that can activate or inhibit genes and pathways involved in colorectal cancer development. As a whole, these studies found that the up-regulated hsa-miR-183-5p and hsa-miR-21-5p, as well as the down-regulated hsa-miR-195-5p and hsa-miR-497-5p, were linked to colorectal cancer development via interactions with the Mismatch Repair pathway and the Wnt, RAS, MAPK, PI3K, TGF-, and p53 signaling pathways [27].

3. Integrated bioinformatics analysis tools and databases

Various integrated bioinformatics databases have been utilized for the identification of prognostic biomarkers in the treatment of various kinds of cancer. Some of which have been enlisted in **Table 2** along with database links. The biomarkers associated with different types of Cancers identified with the help of integrated bioinformatics tools depicted in **Figure 3**.

3.1 Microarray and RNASeq data collection

The microarray data collection is done using the GEO database which refers to Gene Expression Omnibus. It could be easily accessed via online medium using http://www.ncbi.nlm.nih.gov/geo/link. The GEO database is basically being used to obtain high-throughput gene expression profiles of PTC (Papillary thyroid carcinoma) and normal thyroid tissues. Independent datasets are chosen, and they are all based on the specified platforms, including the relevant tissues. As per our review of various studies which are aforementioned in this chapter, various microarray datasets have been collected using the GEO database and then processed with bioinformatics to discover hub genes. Several new technologies have emerged for the analysis of gene expression and for the identification of cancer biomarkers. One such technology is RNASeq technology which is nowadays considered to be the most up to date technology to analyze gene expression. Into this technology, with the use of NGS (Next generation genome sequencer) the gene expression profile analysis carried out. The first stage in the process is to convert the population of RNA to be sequenced into complementary DNA (cDNA) fragments which is present in biological sample (a cDNA library). This is accomplished using reverse transcription, allowing the RNA

S. No.	Name of database	Link/URL
1	Gene Expression Omnibus (GEO)	http://www.ncbi.nlm.nih.gov/geo/
2	GEO2R	http://www.ncbi.nlm.nih.gov/geo/geo2r/
3	DAVID	http://david.abcc.ncifcrf.gov/
4	STRING	http://www.bork.embl-heidelberg.de/STRING/
5	Cytoscape	http://www.cytoscape.org/
6	GEPIA	http://gepia2021.cancer-pku.cn/
7	TGCA	https://tcga-data.nci.nih.gov/tcga/
8	Kaplan–Meier (KM) Plotter	http://kmplot.com/analysis/
9	DIANA-mirPath	http://www.microrna.gr/miRPathv3
10	mirDIP	http://ophid.utoronto.ca/mirDIP
11	GOplot	http://cran.r-project.org/web/packages/GOplot
12	clueGO	http://apps.cytoscape.org/apps/cluego
13	MCODE	http://baderlab.org/Software/MCODE
14	GTEx	https://gtexportal.org
15	Oncomine	http://www.oncomine.org/resource/login.html
16	Human Protein Atlas	www.proteinatlas.org
17	miRWalk	http://mirwalk.uni-hd.de/
18	TargetScan	www.targetscan.org
19	OncomiR	http://www.oncomir.org/oncomir/search_target_miR.html

Table 2.
List of databases used for data mining.

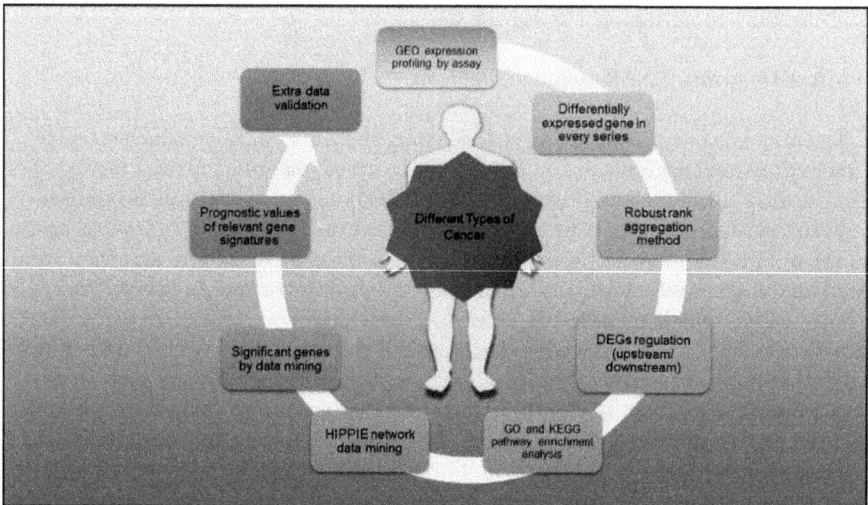

Figure 3.
Mechanistic insight of extraction, construction and identification of biomarkers associated with different kinds of cancers with the help of integrated bioinformatics tools.

to be used in an NGS procedure. After that, the cDNA is fragmented, and adapters are attached to each fragment's end. The functional elements present on adopters which allowed sequencing. The cDNA library is evaluated by NGS after amplification, size selection, clean-up, and quality verification, yielding short sequences that correspond to all or part of the fragment from which it was formed. The extent to which the library is sequenced is determined by the intended use of the output data. Sequencing can be done in one of two ways: single-end or paired-end. Single-read sequencing is a less expensive and faster method of sequencing cDNA fragments from only one end (approximately 1% of the cost of Sanger sequencing). While paired-end approaches are more expensive since they sequence from both ends, but they provide advantages in post-sequencing data reconstruction. After completing the RNA sequencing technology workflow, the data can be matched to a reference genome if one is available, or built from scratch to provide an RNA sequence map that encompasses the transcriptome. A bioinformatics workflow is developed to discover various alternative biomarkers via LC- MS/MS technique (liquid chromatography coupled tandem mass spectrometry). Further, open Mass spectrometry Search Algorithm is used against the customized alternative splicing database along with the preferred cancer plasma proteome for the identification of respective biomarker [50, 51].

3.2 Screening of DEGs

The GEO2R program which could be easily accessed via http://www.ncbi.nlm.nih. gov/geo/geo2r/link, is used for the detection of these differentially expressed genes which are known as DEGs. Further, R package Limma is been utilized to screen out these DEGs.

3.3 Enrichment analysis via GO and KEGG pathway

Followed by the screening of DEGs, the enrichment analysis using GO and KEGG pathway is performed using the database for Annotation, Visualization and Integrated Discovery, commonly known as DAVID database (http://david.abcc.ncifcrf.gov/). This process includes biological processes, cellular components, molecular function and KEGG pathway analysis. Further, the GOplot package of R could be used to display the results of analysis and the pathway analysis results can also be analyzed using the clueGO plug-ins of cytoscape software 3.7.2. [52].

3.4 Construction of the PPI network and analysis of the module

After the enrichment analysis, the PPI network is being built upon using the STRING (http://www.bork.embl-heidelberg.de/STRING/) database which refers to Search Tool for the Retrieval of Interacting Genes/Proteins, to uncover DEG associations based on minimum prescribed interaction scores. Followed by this, using the Cytoscape (http://www.cytoscape.org/) database, the PPI network is then analyzed and visualized. Additionally, MCODE is also one such bioinformatics tool utilized to screen the PPI network's main module.

3.5 Survival analysis and validation of hub gene expression

At last. The Cancer Genome Atlas (https://tcga-data.nci.nih.gov/tcga/), was utilized to examine the association between important gene expression and survival of patients with PTC (Papillary thyroid carcinoma). RNA expression data from hundreds of samples from the TCGA and GTEx projects was analyzed using the Gene Expression Profiling Interactive Analysis tool (GEPIA) (http://gepia2021.cancer-pku. cn/). Additionally Oncomine, Human Protein Atlas, and Kaplan Meier plotter tool databases could also be used to look at the translational and protein expression levels, as well as survival statistics, of DEGs. Apart from this, miRWalk and TargetScan, were used to predict the corresponding change in the expression level of microRNAs in DEGs and the expression profiles were evaluated using OncomiR. Finally, RT-qPCR has been used to confirm the expression of new DEGs. Hence, the constructed biomarkers could be treated as potential candidates for various kinds of Cancers.

4. Challenges and future outlook

The development of biomarkers for early detection cancer screening and therapy monitoring has biological as well as financial hurdles. The majority of existing cancer detection tools only detect late stage or fully grown cancer, not premalignant or early abnormalities that can be resected and treated. Despite the fact that a screening test may detect cancer just at preclinical stage, it is not suitable for follow-up, and hence may miss micro metastases, limiting the benefits of early identification and treatment [53]. Additional barrier to the development of cancer biomarkers is the fact that cancer is a diverse illness, with several biologically distinct phenotypes that respond differently to treatments. Between cells of a single macroscopic tumor, the nature of its heterogeneity can be found. Biomarker development may be hampered by this variability. As a result, developing biomarkers using genomic and proteomic methods could help to solve the variability challenges [3]. An even more issue is that pre-neoplastic lesions are far more common than aggressive malignancies in several organs, such as the prostate and colon [54]. This addresses the possibility of whether any screening strategy should focus solely on early lesions or should additionally consider the tumor's behavior. In the last two decades, detailed and comprehensive knowledge of cancer at the cellular and molecular levels has increased dramatically and exponentially, resulting in significant improvements in the characterization of human tumors, which has catalyzed a shift toward the development of targeted therapies, the foundation of molecular diagnostics [55, 56]. Omics technology may serve as the foundation for the development of novel cancer biomarker and/or panels that have significant advantages over currently utilized biomarkers. Omics has enhanced the number of potential biomarkers such as DNA, RNA, and other protein biomolecules that may be studied. The previous idea of single biomarker discovery has lately been supplanted by multi-biomarker discovery of a panel of genes or proteins, raising the question of whether heterogeneous and complex cancers can have a single fingerprint.

Biomarkers in association with cancer are used in oncology and clinical practice for risk assessment, screening, and diagnosis in combination with other diagnostic methods, and most importantly for determining prognosis and treatment response and/or recurrence. Cancer biomarkers can also help with cancer diagnosis at the molecular level. Clinicians and researchers must have a thorough understanding of the molecular aspects, clinical utility, and reliability of biomarkers in order to determine whether or not a biomarker is clinically useful for patient care and whether or not additional evaluation is required before integration into routine care. Biomarkers, through simplifying the integration of therapies and diagnostics, have the potential to play a key role in the development of customized medicine.

5. Conclusions

Research in the field of cancer-specific biomarkers have provided a promising source of novel diagnostic tools. Various groups have reported that altered cancer-associated biomarkers can be exploited to diagnose and monitor various cancers with greater sensitivity and specificity. Assessment of genomic and transcriptomic biomarkers found to be potentially very sensitive approaches for discriminating between cancerous non-cancerous (benign) conditions. Besides, this one could detect cancers at a much earlier stage by quantitative analysis of potential biomarker associated with specific cancer. Given the possible diagnostic power of genomic, transcriptomic, proteomic, and metabolomic biomarkers, these are currently one of the most promising areas of research in the field of development of cancer prognostic and diagnostics devices.

Author details

Arpana Parihar[1*], Shivani Malviya[2] and Raju Khan[1,3]

1 Microfluidics and MEMS Centre, CSIR-Advanced Materials and Processes Research Institute (AMPRI), Bhopal, India

2 Department of Biochemistry and Genetics, Barkatullah University, Bhopal, Madhya Pradesh, India

3 Academy of Scientific and Innovative Research (AcSIR), CSIR-AMPRI, Bhopal, India

*Address all correspondence to: arpana_parihar@yahoo.com

IntechOpen

References

[1] Bertram JS. The molecular biology of cancer. Molecular Aspects of Medicine. 2000;**21**(6):167-223

[2] Zitvogel L, Tesniere A, Kroemer G. Cancer despite immunosurveillance: Immunoselection and immunosubversion. Nature Reviews Immunology. 2006;**6**(10): 715-727

[3] Wagner PD, Verma M, Srivastava S. Challenges for biomarkers in cancer detection. Annals of the New York Academy of Sciences. 2004;**1022**(1):9-16

[4] Ludwig JA, Weinstein JN. Biomarkers in cancer staging, prognosis and treatment selection. Nature Reviews Cancer. 2005;**5**(11):845-856

[5] Ames BN, Gold LS, Willett WC. The causes and prevention of cancer. Proceedings of the National Academy of Sciences. 1995;**92**(12):5258-5265

[6] Ni M, Liu X, Wu J, Zhang D, Tian J, Wang T, et al. Identification of candidate biomarkers correlated with the pathogenesis and prognosis of non-small cell lung cancer via integrated bioinformatics analysis. Frontiers in Genetics. 2018;**9**. DOI: 10.3389/fgene. 2018.00469

[7] Dai B, Ren L-Q, Han X-Y, Liu D-J. Bioinformatics analysis reveals 6 key biomarkers associated with non-small-cell lung cancer. The Journal of International Medical Research. 2020;**48**(3):1-14. DOI: 10.1177/ 0300060519887637

[8] Cui Y, Hunt A, Li Z, Birkin E, Lane J, Ruge F, et al. Lead DEAD/H box helicase biomarkers with the therapeutic potential identified by integrated bioinformatic approaches in lung cancer.

Computational and Structural Biotechnology Journal. 2021;**19**:261-278

[9] Liao Y, Yin G, Wang X, Zhong P, Fan X, Huang C. Identification of candidate genes associated with the pathogenesis of small cell lung cancer via integrated bioinformatics analysis. Oncology Letters. 2019;**18**(4):3723-3733

[10] Tu H, Wu M, Huang W, Wang L. Screening of potential biomarkers and their predictive value in early stage non-small cell lung cancer: A bioinformatics analysis. Translational Lung Cancer Research. 2019;**8**(6): 797-807

[11] Zhang J, Li D, Zhang Y, Ding Z, Zheng Y, Chen S, et al. Integrative analysis of mRNA and miRNA expression profiles reveals seven potential diagnostic biomarkers for non-small cell lung cancer. Oncology Reports. 2020;**43**(1):99-112

[12] Liu X, Wu J, Zhang D, Bing Z, Tian J, Ni M, et al. Identification of potential key genes associated with the pathogenesis and prognosis of gastric cancer based on integrated bioinformatics analysis. Frontiers in Genetics. 2018;**9**. DOI: 10.3389/fgene.2018.00265

[13] Wang W, He Y, Zhao Q, Zhao X, Li Z. Identification of potential key genes in gastric cancer using bioinformatics analysis. Biomedical Reports. 2020;**12**(4): 178-192

[14] Rong L, Huang W, Tian S, Chi X, Zhao P, Liu F. COL1A2 is a novel biomarker to improve clinical prediction in human gastric cancer: Integrating bioinformatics and meta-analysis. Pathology Oncology Research. 2018; **24**(1):129-134

[15] Miao Y, Sui J, Xu S-Y, Liang G-Y, Pu Y-P, Yin L-H. Comprehensive analysis of a novel four-lncRNA signature as a prognostic biomarker for human gastric cancer. Oncotarget. 2017;**8**(43): 75007-75024

[16] Zhang X, Zhang W, Jiang Y, Liu K, Ran L, Song F. Identification of functional lncRNAs in gastric cancer by integrative analysis of GEO and TCGA data. Journal of Cellular Biochemistry. 2019;**120**(10):17898-17911

[17] Ji Y, Yin Y, Zhang W. Integrated bioinformatic analysis identifies networks and promising biomarkers for hepatitis B virus-related hepatocellular carcinoma. International Journal of Genomics. 2020;**2020**:2061024

[18] Shen B, Li K, Zhang Y. Identification of modules and novel prognostic biomarkers in liver cancer through integrated bioinformatics analysis. FEBS Open Bio. 2020;**10**(11):2388-2403

[19] Li L, Lei Q, Zhang S, Kong L, Qin B. Screening and identification of key biomarkers in hepatocellular carcinoma: Evidence from bioinformatic analysis. Oncology Reports. 2017;**38**(5):2607-2618

[20] Wang CCN, Li CY, Cai J-H, Sheu PC-Y, Tsai JJP, Wu M-Y, et al. Identification of prognostic candidate genes in breast cancer by integrated bioinformatic analysis. Journal of Clinical Medicine. 2019;**8**(8):1160

[21] Wu M, Li Q, Wang H. Identification of novel biomarkers associated with the prognosis and potential pathogenesis of breast cancer via integrated bioinformatics analysis. Technology in Cancer Research & Treatment. 2021;**20**:1-16. DOI: 10.1177/1533033821992081

[22] Cai Y, Mei J, Xiao Z, Xu B, Jiang X, Zhang Y, et al. Identification of five hub genes as monitoring biomarkers for breast cancer metastasis in silico. Hereditas. 2019;**156**(1). DOI: 10.1186/s41065-019-0096-6

[23] Wu J, Lv Q, Huang H, Zhu M, Meng D. Screening and identification of key biomarkers in inflammatory breast cancer through integrated bioinformatic analyses. Genetic Testing and Molecular Biomarkers. 2020;**24**(8):484-491

[24] Chen L, Lu D, Sun K, Xu Y, Hu P, Li X, et al. Identification of biomarkers associated with diagnosis and prognosis of colorectal cancer patients based on integrated bioinformatics analysis. Gene. 2019;**692**:119-125

[25] Dai M, Chen X, Mo S, Li J, Huang Z, Huang S, et al. Meta-signature LncRNAs serve as novel biomarkers for colorectal cancer: Integrated bioinformatics analysis, experimental validation and diagnostic evaluation. Scientific Reports. 2017;**7**(1). DOI: 10.1038/srep46572

[26] Sun Z, Liu C, Cheng SY. Identification of four novel prognosis biomarkers and potential therapeutic drugs for human colorectal cancer by bioinformatics analysis. Journal of Biomedical Research. 2021;**35**(1):21

[27] Falzone L, Scola L, Zanghì A, Biondi A, Di Cataldo A, Libra M, et al. Integrated analysis of colorectal cancer microRNA datasets: Identification of microRNAs associated with tumor development. Aging (Albany NY). 2018;**10**(5):1000-1014

[28] van Zandwijk N. New methods for early diagnosis of lung cancer. Lung Cancer. 2002;**38**(1):S9-S11

[29] Torre LA, Bray F, Siegel RL, Ferlay J, Lortet-Tieulent J, Jemal A. Global cancer statistics, 2012. CA: a Cancer Journal for Clinicians. 2015;**65**(2):87-108

[30] Ferro A, Peleteiro B, Malvezzi M, Bosetti C, Bertuccio P, Levi F, et al. Worldwide trends in gastric cancer mortality (1980-2011), with predictions to 2015, and incidence by subtype. European Journal of Cancer. 2014;**50**(7): 1330-1344

[31] Li R, Zhuang C, Jiang S, Du N, Zhao W, Tu L, et al. ITGBL1 predicts a poor prognosis and correlates EMT phenotype in gastric cancer. Journal of Cancer. 2017;**8**(18):3764-3773

[32] Van Cutsem E, Sagaert X, Topal B, Haustermans K, Prenen H. Gastric cancer. Lancet. 2016;**388**(10060): 2654-2664

[33] Chau I. Checkpoint inhibition: An ATTRACTION in advanced gastric cancer? Lancet. 2017;**390**(10111): 2418-2419

[34] Kang M-H, Choi H, Oshima M, Cheong J-H, Kim S, Lee JH, et al. Author Correction: Estrogen-related receptor gamma functions as a tumor suppressor in gastric cancer. Nature Communications. 2018;**9**(1):3599

[35] Wang Z, Chen G, Wang Q, Lu W, Xu M. Identification and validation of a prognostic 9-genes expression signature for gastric cancer. Oncotarget. 2017; **8**(43):73826-73836

[36] Cancer Genome Atlas Research Network. Comprehensive molecular characterization of gastric adeno-carcinoma. Nature. 2014;**513**(7517): 202-209

[37] Sun M, Song H, Wang S, Zhang C, Zheng L, Chen F, et al. Integrated analysis identifies microRNA-195 as a suppressor of Hippo-YAP pathway in colorectal cancer. Journal of Hematology & Oncology. 2017;**10**(1). DOI: 10.1186/s13045-017-0445-8

[38] Sun C, Yuan Q, Wu D, Meng X, Wang B. Identification of core genes and outcome in gastric cancer using bioinformatics analysis. Oncotarget. 2017;**8**(41):70271-70280

[39] Song E, Song W, Ren M, Xing L, Ni W, Li Y, et al. Identification of potential crucial genes associated with carcinogenesis of clear cell renal cell carcinoma. Journal of Cellular Biochemistry. 2018;**119**(7):5163-5174

[40] Wu J, Zhu P, Lu T, Du Y, Wang Y, He L, et al. The long non-coding RNA LncHDAC2 drives the self-renewal of liver cancer stem cells via activation of Hedgehog signaling. Journal of Hepatology. 2019;**70**(5):918-929

[41] Siegel RL, Miller KD, Jemal A. Cancer statistics, 2018. CA: A Cancer Journal for Clinicians. 2018;**68**(1):7-30

[42] Bai Y, Long J, Liu Z, Lin J, Huang H, Wang D, et al. Comprehensive analysis of a ceRNA network reveals potential prognostic cytoplasmic lncRNAs involved in HCC progression. Journal of Cellular Physiology. 2019;**234**(10):18837-18848

[43] Bhikoo R, Srinivasa S, Yu T-C, Moss D, Hill AG. Systematic review of breast cancer biology in developing countries (part 2): Asian subcontinent and South East Asia. Cancers (Basel). 2011;**3**(2):2382-2401

[44] Waks AG, Winer EP. Breast cancer treatment: A review. JAMA. 2019; **321**(3):288-300 19323

[45] Tang J, Kong D, Cui Q, Wang K, Zhang D, Gong Y, et al. Prognostic genes of breast cancer identified by gene co-expression network analysis. Frontiers in Oncology. 2018;**8**:374

[46] Yuan L, Chen L, Qian K, Qian G, Wu CL, Wang X, et al. Coexpression

network analysis identified six hub genes in association with progression and prognosis in human clear cell renal cell carcinoma (ccRCC). Genomics Data. 2017;**14**:132-140

[47] Li J, Zhou D, Qiu W, Shi Y, Yang J-J, Chen S, et al. Application of weighted gene co-expression network analysis for data from paired design. Scientific Reports. 2018;**8**(1):1-8. DOI: 10.1038/s41598-017-18705-z

[48] Kolligs FT. Diagnostics and epidemiology of colorectal cancer. Visceral Medicine. 2016;**32**(3):158-164

[49] Coppedè F. Genetic and epigenetic biomarkers for diagnosis, prognosis and treatment of colorectal cancer. World Journal of Gastroenterology. 2014;**20**(4):943

[50] Zhang F, Deng CK, Wang M, Deng B, Barber R, Huang G. Identification of novel alternative splicing biomarkers for breast cancer with LC/MS/MS and RNA-Seq. BMC Bioinformatics. 2020;**21**(9):1-7

[51] Yamada A, Yu P, Lin W, Okugawa Y, Boland CR, Goel A. A RNA-Sequencing approach for the identification of novel long non-coding RNA biomarkers in colorectal cancer. Scientific Reports. 2018;**8**(1):1

[52] Yang J, Wang F, Zhong S, Chen B. Identification of hub genes with prognostic values in multiple myeloma by bioinformatics analysis. Hematology. 2021;**26**(1):453-459

[53] Pollak MN, Foulkes WD. Challenges to cancer control by screening. Nature Reviews Cancer. 2003;**3**(4):297-303

[54] Neugut AI, Jacobson JS, Rella VA. Prevalence and incidence of colorectal adenomas and cancer in asymptomatic

persons. Gastrointestinal Endoscopy Clinics of North America. 1997;**7**(3):387-399

[55] Diamandis EP. Towards identification of true cancer biomarkers. BMC Medicine. 2014;**12**(1):1-4

[56] Kulasingam V, Pavlou MP, Diamandis EP. Integrating high-throughput technologies in the quest for effective biomarkers for ovarian cancer. Nature Reviews Cancer. 2010;**10**(5):371-378

Chapter 5

The Clinical Usefulness of Prostate Cancer Biomarkers: Current and Future Directions

Donovan McGrowder, Lennox Anderson-Jackson,

Lowell Dilworth, Shada Mohansingh, Melisa Anderson Cross,

Sophia Bryan, Fabian Miller, Cameil Wilson-Clarke,

Chukwuemeka Nwokocha, Ruby Alexander-Lindo

and Shelly McFarlane

Abstract

Worldwide, prostate cancer (PCa) is the leading cause of morbidity and cancer-related mortality in men. The pathogenesis of PCa is complex and involves abnormal genetic changes, abrogation of cell growth with heterogeneous progression and predictive subgroups. In the last two decades there have been the exploration and development of molecular and genetic biomarkers for PCa due to limitations of traditional serum biomarkers such as prostate specific antigen (PSA) in screening and diagnosis. These biomarkers could possibly differentiate between PCa and benign prostatic hyperplasia (BPH) patients, and healthy controls as well as assist with prognosis, risk stratification and clinical decision-making. Such molecular biomarkers include serum (PHI and 4K score), urine (PCA3 and SelectMDx), and tumor tissue (Oncoytype DX, Decipher and Prolarix). microRNAs (miRNAs) deregulation where there is increased or decreased expression levels, constitute prospective non-invasive molecular biomarkers for the diagnosis and prognosis of PCa. There are also other emerging molecular biomarkers such as exosomal miRNAs and proteins that are in various stages of development and clinical research. This review is intended to provide a wide-ranging appraisal of the literature on current and emerging PCa biomarkers with robust evidence to afford their application in clinical research and by extension routine clinical practice.

Keywords: prostate, cancer, biomarkers, diagnosis, prognosis, molecular, emerging, clinical

1. Introduction

Prostate cancer (PCa) is a complex condition characterized by varying clinical behaviors ranging from indolence to metastatic disease states. Globally, PCa was

IntechOpen

the second most prevalent cancer and the fifth major cause of cancer-related deaths among men in 2020. Strikingly, about 1.4 million new cancer cases and 375,000 deaths were attributable to PCa in 2020 [1]. Approximately one in nine men will be diagnosed with PCa in their lifetime [2]. Increased widespread screening using prostate specific antigen (PSA) mirrors the epidemic rise of PCa with geographic variability. However, since the advent of PSA screening, mortality rates have significantly declined [3]. The incidence of PCa in countries with low Human Development Index (HDI) was about three times lower than those with high HDI, 11.3 vs. 37.5 per 100,000 persons respectively [1]. The highest incidences were reported in the Caribbean, Northern and Western Europe, Australia/New Zealand, Southern Africa and North American regions [1]. The Caribbean and Sub-Saharan Africa accounted for the highest mortality rates [1]. There is mounting evidence that PCa disproportionately affects men of African ancestry. In the United States, African American men are 58% more likely to be affected by PCa with a 144% higher risk of PCa-specific mortality than their Caucasian counterparts [4]. The established risk factors of the disease include: increasing age, race and family history of PCa [5]. PSA is currently the most widely used screening tool for PCa indication, but a number of studies have highlighted its failure to discriminate between indolence and more aggressive forms of the disease. The low positive predictive value (PPV) of PSA has led to over-diagnosis of low-grade cancer and complications from unnecessary biopsies [6] as no cancer is detected on approximately 50% of biopsies [7].

Total prostate specific antigen (tPSA) is not very sensitive in detecting early PCa, and being cancer-specific as there are elevated levels in prostatitis, urogenital infections, BPH and transurethral manipulations. False positive results leads to increased rate of over-diagnosis, further expensive diagnostic evaluations and invasive procedures, and possibly over-treatment [8]. There are also false negatives particularly in the 'gray zone' (with tPSA values 4–10 ng/mL) resulting in undiagnosed PCa [9]. Furthermore, there is the absence of a linear correlation between serum tPSA and metastatic PCa as well as staging [10].

In order to increase the diagnostic utility of PSA for PCa, new biomarker such as Prostate Health Index (PHI), four K (4K) score and prostate cancer antigen 3 (PCA3) have become available. These tests decrease the number of needless prostate biopsies, provide valuable information on tumor aggressiveness and aid in the selection of PCa patients for radical therapy or active surveillance [11]. Genomic techniques have permitted the accessibility of novel genetic biomarkers such as transmembrane serine protease 2 (TMPRSS2:ERG fusion gene), Oncotype DX, Decipher and ProMark which stratify the risk of aggressive PCa and aid decision-making by providing information on diagnosis, prognosis and treatment [12].

This article seeks to review current advances in the development and availability of PCa biomarkers and their precise indications for diagnostic, prognostic, predictive and use in monitoring therapeutic response. Current and emerging biomarkers are appraised including their possible integration into medical practice and enhancing the clinical management of PCa.

2. Method of article selection

2.1 Study eligibility criteria

A literature search and review of recent publications in PubMed, Google Scholar, Embase and Cochrane library relating to the clinical utility of PCa biomarkers were conducted. The search examined all relevant published studies up to January 20, 2022. The studies included in this review were published in peer-reviewed journals, written in English, and reported medical as well as scientific findings. Also, pertinent data that were extracted from published studies include: authors, year of publication and study design and population. Information from the articles concerning molecular biomarkers of PCa used for screening, diagnosis, prognosis, risk stratification and therapeutic tools were reviewed and documented.

3. Results

3.1 Blood-based prostate cancer biomarkers

3.1.1 Prostate specific antigen

Currently, the diagnosis of PCa is based on the results of digital rectal examination (DRE), trans-rectal ultrasound guided biopsy and PSA assay [13]. The aim of utilizing the least invasive methods has led to increased use of PSA as a biomarker. However, the use of PSA is limited by its low specificity, which in turn results in over-diagnosis of PCa followed by unnecessary biopsies and associated potential complications [14]. In the detection of PCa, serum total PSA (tPSA) > 4.0 ng/mL has a 94% sensitivity but only a 20% specificity, which makes the test unsuitable for screening [15]. There are also several limitations to PSA testing in the detection of high-grade PCa, with data from the Prostate Cancer Prevention Trial (PCPT) indicating that in order to achieve a sensitivity of 83.4%, a tPSA threshold of 1.1 ng/mL is required. However, the corresponding specificity was only 39.9% [16]. Since tPSA may be elevated in conditions other than PCa, only about 25% of men with elevated tPSA will be diagnosed, while there is still a 10% chance of patients with tPSA <1.0 ng/mL developing the disease [17]. In light of these limitations, several variations to the PSA assay have been implemented to increase specificity of the test. These includes: free PSA (fPSA), PSA velocity, free-to-total PSA (fPSA/tPSA) ratio and PSA density (PSAD). In addition to these PSA variation tests, prostate specific antibodies may also be useful in selecting men for biopsies especially since localized PCa may not present with symptoms [18].

PSA is typically found in the bound or free form. Bound PSA refers to PSA found complexed to protease inhibitors like alpha-1-antichymotrypsin, while fPSA which is found unbound is mostly inactive and associated with BPH as opposed to PCa [19]. A fraction of fPSA can however be active as such tPSA, refers to any of the active or inactive forms found in serum [20]. In light of these variations in PSA, specific assays targeting precise fractions have been developed. Bound or complexed PSA is found to be elevated in malignancies while the calculation of fPSA/tPSA ratio gives values that are normally lower in men with PCa [21, 22]. The fPSA/tPSA ratio is indicative of %fPSA and has been shown to increase the accuracy of PSA use in detection of PCa [23] (**Table 1**).

3.1.1.1 PSA use in detection of prostate cancer

Initial studies indicated that PCa was more likely with <25% fPSA at a sensitivity of 95%. However, subsequent similar studies have yielded unreliable results owing to the instability of fPSA making it a somewhat an unreliable marker on its own [54, 55]. This could be as a result of storage conditions as subsequent studies indicated that the stability of tPSA and fPSA levels in serum did not depreciate

Biomarker tests	Molecular markers	Specimen	Outcome	References
Prostate specific antigen (PSA)	tPSA, fPSA, %fPSA	Serum/ plasma	Screening, diagnosis	[13, 20, 24, 25]
Prostate Cancer Antigen-3 gene (PCA3)	Ratio PCA3 mRNA/ PSA mRNA × 1000	Urine	Diagnosis, prognosis	[13, 26–28]
Select MDx	HOXC6, DLX1, tPSA, clinical parameters	Urine	Diagnosis, prognosis, risk stratification	[29, 30]
K score	tPSA, fPSA, intact PSA, human kallikrein-related peptidase 2	Serum/ plasma	Diagnosis, prediction	[31, 32]
The Decipher	22 RNA genes	Biopsy tissue	Risk stratification, therapy decision making	[33–44]
Oncotype DX Genomic Prostate Score (GPS)	12 cancer related genes, & 5 reference genes	Biopsy tissue	Prediction, risk stratification, therapy decision making	[41, 43–48]
ConfirmMDX	DNA methylation of GSTP1, APC, & RASSF1 gene	Biopsy prostate cores	Prediction (repeat biopsies)	[49–51]
The ProMark	8 proteomic biomarkers	Biopsy tissue	Prediction, risk assessment	[52, 53]

Table 1.
Summary of currently available biomarkers for use in prostate cancer screening, diagnosis, detection or stratification.

significantly after 10 years storage at −80°C [29]. Other studies on tPSA and %fPSA have shown conflicting data as seen in the case of a 2009 study by Omar et al. [24]. Here, %fPSA values were high in patients diagnosed with PCa compared with BPH, while tPSA was found to be a better serum marker for diagnosing PCa in that cohort. However, a Chinese study highlighted that for men in the PSA gray zone, the inclusion of %fPSA will improve the diagnostic accuracy for PCa, and high grade PCa compared with only tPSA [25].

Clinical usefulness of PSA variations appears to be age-specific as a study comprising patients over 60 years old showed that tPSA outperformed %fPSA and therefore had the higher predictive value for detecting high grade carcinoma [20]. Moreover, an Asian study suggested that age-specific ranges for tPSA, fPSA and %fPSA could be considered in the diagnostic workup of PCa. Results from that study highlighted that there was a gradual increase in reference interval for tPSA and fPSA peaking at 7.73 and 2.41 ng/ mL respectively for those over 80 years old. The researchers also reported that reference intervals for %fPSA were ≥16.0 for 21–50 years and ≥13.0 for males over 50 years old [56]. In a South American study of over 17,000 men, %fPSA value of <15 as an indication for biopsy was shown to increase the rate of PCa detection in patients with normal DRE results and serum tPSA of 2.5–4.0 ng/mL [17].

Although the results vary with different studies, the PSA parameters mentioned seem to have significant predictive values in PCa screening and should be utilized based on the cohort along with other clinical factors in assessing PCa. This is in line with the conclusion by some researchers that especially within the gray zone, a multivariate model is a useful tool in diagnosing PCa, and clinically significant PCa while reducing unnecessary biopsies in the process [18].

3.1.2 Prostate cancer antigen-3 gene

The thrust to discovering other biomarkers of PCa is based on the limitations that exist with regard to utilization of PSA or other invasive investigatory methods. Given the complications associated with PCa detection and treatment, the ultimate goal from a clinical perspective appears to be discovery of biomarkers that more accurately predict PCa and clinically significant disease prior to biopsy in an attempt to reduce the number of unnecessary biopsy requests [57].

Over time, some molecular biomarkers have been developed with emphasis placed on those that are capable of predicting disease aggressiveness that will lead to improved guidance for treatment modalities. Some of these markers are serum while others are urine-based.

To date, the most commonly used urinary biomarker of PCa is PCA3 otherwise referred to as Differential Display clone 3 (DD3). It is conventionally assessed in urine post prostate massage to derive the maximum number of prostatic cells, and was the first urinary RNA biomarker approved by the Food and Drug Administration (FDA) in 2012 [58]. Discovered around 1995 by researchers in the USA and The Netherlands, PCA3 is non-coding messenger RNA from chromosome 9q21-22, consisting of four exons and three introns and is over-expressed in most tested PCa tissues [59–61]. Additionally, PCA3 is over-expressed in prostate tumor tissue compared with other benign prostate disorders [13, 26]. It therefore aids in improving the accuracy of PSA with regards to management of early PCa and as such, approval was granted by some developed countries for its use as a molecular marker in the diagnostic workup of PCa owing to improved specificity for PCa over PSA [62, 63]. In fact, the use of PCA3 in tandem with other molecular markers including transmembrane serine protease 2 (TMPRSS2)-ERG, human kallikrein 2, and miRNA-141 was found to have significant clinical utility by way of increasing specificity, and in predicting PCa especially in the PSA gray area of 4–10 ng/mL [13].

Assessment of urinary PCA3 can be done by way of the quantitative real-time PCR (qRT-PCR) reaction followed by generation of a PCA3 score utilizing the ratio of PCA3 to tPSA [64, 65]. In utilizing this method, a negative biopsy result is 4.5 times more likely in men with a score of <25 compared with those with a score >25 [66]. Importantly, low-volume and low-grade disease are seen in men with low PCA3 scores [67]. A study on 407 high risk PCa patients indicated that PCA3 has clinical useful-ness as a formidable prognostic indicator of tumor aggressiveness and was associated with higher PCA3 scores [27]. A high PCA3 score was also shown to be a good predic-tor of a positive PCa diagnosis and displayed greater accuracy than fPSA and tPSA in this regard (**Table 1**) [27, 28]. These results are in contrast to other studies indicating that the PPV of tPSA for diagnosing PCa was only 25% which directly increases the chances of obtaining false positive results in a quarter of cases and consequently a high chance of unnecessary biopsy in 75% of cases [57, 68, 69].

3.1.3 Prostate health index

The prostate health index (PHI) is a modern test that utilized PSA in accelerating the diagnosis of PCa. This particular biomarker has been sanctioned and approved in the United States, Europe and Australia. Studies conducted globally have depicted the reliably of PHI as a biomarker that outclasses its individual components for the prognostication of overall and high-grade PCa on biopsy [70]. This represent PCa with Gleason score (GS) that is ≥7 [71].

In utilizing PHI as a biomarker, it allows for the combination of the tPSA, fPSA and [−2]proPSA (p2PSA) into a formula to produce a single result that can be used to assist in clinical decision-making of PCa. Such PHI formula computation is ([−2] proPSA/fPSA) × $\sqrt{PSA}$ and demonstrates the possibility of clinically significant PCa in men with elevated tPSA and p2PSA while the fPSA is lower [70].

In men that possesses a tPSA between 4 and 10 ng/mL, PHI may be useful in establishing PCa in conjunction with a prostate biopsy. Interestingly, a low possibility of PCa outcome on biopsy is supplementary to small PHI results, while an elevated possibility of PCa outcome on biopsy is directly related to elevated PHI. Different medical considerations or family history of PCa are dominant factors in the management process as it relates to the appropriate PHI value [70, 72, 73].

A huge study was conducted in the USA in 2011 by Catalona et al. The study aimed to demonstrate the diagnostic capability of PHI for PCa recognition in a populace of 892 men with normal DRE, tPSA levels between 2 and 10 ng/mL and a prostate biopsy [73]. Interestingly, based on the PHI reference intervals, a value of 49 was obtained for prostate biopsies that were positive, while 34 was obtained for biopsies that were considered negative. This demonstrates a superior sensitivity and specificity in the diagnosis of PCa, and also differentiating PCa on biopsy compared with tPSA. Although the PHI test has been approved by the FDA only in the tPSA range of 4–10 ng/mL, PHI performed well in the 2–10 ng/mL range [74].

A large multicenter research involving approximately 5543 participants using the bivariate mixed-effect model was conducted by Zhang et al. from 2011 to 2019 to assess the medical significance of PHI in detecting PCa. The results obtained showed the likely sensitivity of PHI for diagnosing PCa of 0.75 and a specificity of 0.69. A value of 0.78 was obtained for the pooled area under the curve (AUC) and the diagnostic odds ratio (OR) was 6.73. The researchers also found that the diagnostic accurateness of PHI for PCa was greater in Asian compared with Caucasian populations (0.83 vs. 0.76). Based on the overall results the authors suggested that PHI has a modest diagnostic accurateness for detecting PCa [75].

Moreover, in a small study of 58 Asian patients with tPSA of 4–10 ng/mL who undertook transrectal ultrasound-guided prostatic biopsy, 18 cases had PCa and the AUC for this biomarker was 0.774. The sensitivity of PHI was 90% with a specificity of 27.5% which was the highest among the group of biomarkers including tPSA, PSAD and %fPSA. The authors suggested that PHI improves the accuracy of predicting PCa and decrease avoidable prostate biopsy [76]. These results are in consonance with another recent study involving 140 Korean patients that underwent prostate biopsy of which there were 63 cases of PCa. The AUC for PHI in the overall group was 0.76 (which was higher than tPSA, fPSA, %fPSA) and in the sub-group with GS ≥ 7, a value of 0.87 was obtained. PHI was a strong independent prognosticator of PCa particularly for the presence and aggressiveness (GS ≥ 7) of the disease, and its application could prevent a substantial amount of unnecessary prostate biopsies [77]. Furthermore, there are other recent studies that have demonstrated that PHI is more specific than tPSA in PCa detection [78] and a better predictor than %fPSA in detecting PCa at prostate biopsy [79].

3.1.4 Four K score

4K score test incorporates the measurement of four biomarkers: tPSA, fPSA, intact PSA, and human kallikrein-related peptidase 2 combined in an algorithm with the patient's clinical information such as age, previous biopsy and DRE to generate the percentage risk (<1% to >95%) for aggressive metastatic PCa with GS ≥ 7 on biopsy [31]. The 4K score test is usually conducted following a previous abnormal DRE or tPSA [31] and supports clinical decision making to determine whether a biopsy should be done. The 4K score has been found to predict high-grade metastatic PCa and estimates an individual's risk of having the disease that spreads to distant organs within 10 years [32]. This was supported by a multi-institutional prospective trial conducted in the United States among 144 men which sought to determine the association between previous 4K score, staging and grading of PCa at radical prostatectomy. It found that higher 4K scores were significantly associated with worse grades and aggressive histology. There was a higher median 4K score among PCa patients with cancer not confined to the prostate when compared with organ-confined cancer [36% (IQR 19, 58)] vs. [19% (IQR 9, 35)], (p = 0.002) [80].

In a clinical study involving 611 patients the 4K score test led to a 65% reduction in unnecessary biopsies [31]. There was also a strong association between high risk 4K score and a greater possibility of having a prostate biopsy. Similarly, another study with a population of 1012 men reported that the 4K score was useful in identifying candidates for biopsies with GS ≥ 7 and could narrow the gap of unnecessary biopsies by 30–58% [7]. However, the researchers highlighted that about 1.3–4.7% of men with aggressive disease may experience a delay in diagnosis using the 4K score [7]. Moreover, a retrospective study performed on 946 men of different racial ethnicities with elevated tPSA levels and a previous biopsy demonstrated that the 4K score had a higher discriminatory index for high-grade PCa compared with the conventional tPSA, DRE, age and PCPT calculator [31]. The researchers showed that among African American men, the detection of metastatic PCa using the 4K score test was significantly enhanced over the use of tPSA with an AUC of 0.80 versus 0.67. Additionally, it was found that the 4K score test would be able to identify 88% of aggressive cancers while reducing 42% of unnecessary biopsies [81].

3.2 Urine-based prostate cancer biomarkers

3.2.1 TMPRSS2-ERG fusion and PCA3

In a similar way to PCA3, a transmembrane serine protease 2 (TMPRSS2)-ERG fusion gene can be detected in urine post-DRE [82]. Various biomarkers are released in urine which may become enriched with prostate material upon manipulation of the prostate gland during a DRE [83]. A TMPRSS2-ERG gene fusion score is comparable to PSA mRNA quantity, in which the latter is currently being used as the gold standard test for PCa. TMPRSS2-ERG fusion gene is a genetic rearrangement of the androgen-regulated trans-membrane protease, serine 2 (TMPRSS2) gene and the ERG (erythroblast transformation-specific; ETS)-related gene. ERG is an oncogene and is a part of the family of transcription factors. TMPRSS2-ERG gene fusion is expressed specifically in PCa and is the most prevalent known type of PCa-specific gene alterations [84, 85]. There are two mechanisms by which TMPRSS2-ERG gene fusion may occur, either by chromosomal translocation or interstitial deletion; the latter being the more predominant mechanism in which approximately 2.8 Mb genetic material may be lost due to occurrence of this event [86–89]. A study reported that the deletion type fusion was found to be highest among African American patients, followed by Caucasians and no significant differences have been seen in Asian populations regarding either type [89]. Targeted inhibition of the TMPRSS2-ERG fusion gene or its gene fusion transcripts could possibly serve as a treatment strategy in the future, thereby resulting in favorable outcomes for PCa patients.

Gene fusion of TMPRSS2 and ERG has been shown to result in an overexpression of ERG. ERG has been shown to play a vital role in cell growth, differentiation, and apoptosis [90]. It is possible that overexpression of ERG triggers a downstream cascade of events that lead to the onset and progression of PCa. Hence, TMPRSS2-ERG gene fusion maybe seen as an early phenomenon that takes place in the development of PCa. TMPRSS2-ERG gene fusion has been detected in 40–70% of PCa patients [88]. The frequency of TMPRSS2-ERG gene fusion has been reported to be greatest among Caucasian Americans (50%), followed by African Americans (31%) and Asians (18.5%) respectively [89].

TMPRSS2-ERG and PCA3 are two of the most studied urine biomarkers with PCA3 having received FDA approval. TMPRSS2-ERG and PCA3 in post-DRE urine for the detection of PCa at biopsy showed significant improvement over PSA [85, 91, 92]. When a Mi-Prostate Score for post-DRE urine, was utilized it was reported that TMPRSS2-ERG had a low sensitivity of 24.3–37.0%. However, the fusion gene had a specificity of 93% and a PPV of 94%. Combination of TMPRSS2-ERG with serum tPSA (a cut-off value of 10 ng/mL) and urinary PCA3, greatly improves the accuracy of diagnosing PCa, from a study that reported a sensitivity of 80% and a specificity of 90% [93]. TMPRSS2-ERG gene fusion test also gives information about a risk assessment for aggressive PCa [94].

It was reported in a study that TMPRSS2-ERG gene fusions showed a significant association with a GS $\geq$7 and PCa-related deaths. When TMPRSS2-ERG and PCA3 were combined with the PCPT risk calculator, the information provided may aid physicians in deciding whether a patient with high serum tPSA will need urgent biopsy [91, 94]. Analyzing ERG mRNA in post-DRE urine in a study cohort of 237 men, a predictive accuracy for AUC of 0.80 was reported for PCa diagnosis in Caucasian men having tPSA levels $\leq$4.0 ng/mL [92]. Studies have supported the combined use of TMPRSS2-ERG and PCA3 in clinical practice to help in reducing the number of prostate biopsies [95]. With this in mind, Kohaar et al. concluded that the data from cumulated studies suggest that when TMPRSS2-ERG and PCA3 are combined along with serum tPSA there were improvements in the detection of aggressive PCa (GS $\geq$7) on initial biopsy with a 42% reduction in unwarranted biopsies [85, 91].

3.2.2 SelectMDx (DLX1, HOXC6)

The SelectMDx test is a urine-based gene expression assay. This assay measures the mRNA levels of two biomarkers, distal-less homeobox 1 (DLX1) and homeobox C6 (HOXC6) using qRT-PCR in post DRE urine [96]. Kallikrein serine protease (KLK3) gene which codes for PSA is used as an internal control for this assay. The test was performed on patients who have risk factors for PCa and were being considered for prostate biopsy. DLX1 and HOXC6 are believed to be involved in the onset of PCa and are both associated with high grade disease [95]. In a study using PCa cell lines, it was found that HOXC6, a transcriptional factor when suppressed, caused a reduction in cell viability and induced apoptosis [97, 98]. In another study investigating the role of DLX1, a protein coding gene, it was reported that DLX1 promoted growth, migration and colony formation of cancer cells [97, 99].

The SelectMDx assay is not a "standalone" test and so incorporates clinical factors such as age, tPSA, prostate volume and DRE findings to estimate the percent likelihood of detecting PCa and high-grade (GS $\geq$ 7) disease upon prostate biopsy. Leyten et al. [30] first identified that a three gene panel of HOXC6, DLX1 and

Tudor domain-containing protein 1 (TDRD1) was able to show higher accuracy (AUC = 0.77) for the detection of clinically significant PCa (csPCa) compared with tPSA (AUC = 0.72) and PCA3 (AUC = 0.68) tests respectively. In follow-up prospective studies, focus was placed on the urinary mRNA levels of HOXC6 and DLX1 genes. Using a large cohort (n = 905), the expression of DLX1 and HOXC6 gave an AUC of 0.76, a sensitivity of 91%, a specificity 36%, a NPV of 94% and PPV of 27% for the prediction of high-grade PCa (**Table 1**) [100]. It was seen that when SelectMDX was combined with clinical factors such as tPSA, PSAD, family history and history of prostate biopsy, the risk stratification of high-grade PCa and biopsy decisions maybe improved as the AUC was 0.90 in identifying high-grade PCa (GS ≥ 7) [100].

In a more recent validation study by Haese et al. [101], the data showed high sensitivity and NPV in detecting csPCa when investigating urinary HOXC6 and DLX1 mRNA levels. These results were combined with patient age, DRE and tPSA levels less than 10 ng/mL which gave an AUC of 0.82, sensitivity 89%, specificity 53% and NPV 95% [102]. Haese et al. [102] concluded that the data supported using the SelectMDx test to aid in decision-making around prostate biopsies. Furthermore, Govers et al. [101] conducted a study on the healthcare cost using SelectMDx for PCa in four European countries. From the results of the study, it was reported that quality-adjusted life years (QALYS) could be gained and that the use of SelectMDx may have favorable economic outcomes for patients at initial PCa diagnosis. Currently, SelectMDx is only available through companies that received CLIA (Clinical Laboratory Improvement Amendments)-approval [102].

3.3 Tissue-based prostate cancer biomarkers

3.3.1 Oncotype DX Genomic Prostate Score

Oncotype DX Genomic Prostate Score (GPS) is considered a molecular biomarker that was established to aid in the prognostication of PCa in men with intermediary possibility of the disease. This particular biomarker is based on 17 genes GPS. This can be further explained where 12 of the genes referred to as qRT-PCR genes are responsible in identifying growth linked to PCa, while the remaining five genes are responsible for demonstrating stromal response, androgen signaling, cellular organization, and proliferation, thereby achieving a computational formula system that resulted in the GPS [103]. This particular Oncotype DX GPS assay measures mRNA expression of the 17 genes accountable for neoplasm progression and was established and reviewed in approximately 4500 patients [104].

A study was conducted to identify and authenticate a biopsy-based 17-gene GPS signature by investigating 732 candidate genes in their clinical utility to predict PCa mortality, adverse pathology and clinical recurrence. The GPS predicted high-grade PCa and clinical recurrence notwithstanding multi-focality and heterogeneity. The authors suggested that the GPS test assist patients in making knowledgeable decisions concerning immediate therapy or active surveillance [103]. In another study, Cullen et al. assessed the association of the 17-gene GPS with clinical recurrence in 431 men with clinically low to intermediate risk PCa. GPS results (scale 0–100) were obtained for 402 PCa patients and it predicted time to metastases and biochemical recurrence. GPS was significantly associated with adverse pathology (OR = 3.3 per 20 GPS) and the predictive outcomes were similar for Caucasian and African American men [43]. Recently, the same authors performed a multicenter comparison of 17-gene Oncotype DX® GPS in Caucasian (n = 1144) and African American (n = 201) men diagnosed with clinically localized PCa. The GPS scores were the same between the two racial groups showing corresponding predictive outcomes, and using a multivariate model, biochemical recurrence and adverse pathology was significantly associated with the GPS assay (**Table 1**) [44]. Supporting evidence of Oncotype DX GPS as an independent predictor of adverse pathology in the two racial groups was provided by Murphy et al. [45] using PCa patients (96 African American and 76 European American men) from two multi-institutional observational studies.

There are other studies such as that performed by Kornberg et al. [46] which found that higher GPS in PCa patients who undertook radical prostatectomy following active surveillance is associated with greater risk of adverse pathology and biochemical recurrence. Lynch et al. [47] reported that GPS testing was a valuable tool in risk stratification among PCa patients and those who are low risk are more likely to make the decision to adopt active surveillance. Notably, Chang et al. posited that the deployment of GPS was worthwhile in guiding decisions regarding therapy in patients with early stage PCa compared with active surveillance [48]. The finding that the GPS test is associated with long-term outcomes such as PCa-specific mortality and distant metastases is also worth mentioning [105]. However, in a recent study there was no significant association of the GPS test with adverse pathology after initial period of neither active surveillance nor improvement in risk stratification for adverse pathology versus the use of only clinical variables [106].

3.3.2 The Decipher

The Decipher, a molecular biomarker is categorized as a genomic assessment, established by GenomeDx Biosciences in Vancouver, Canada. This particular test evaluates the expression signature of approximately 22 RNA genes that demonstrates the prognostication and progression of PCa. Among the various genes group, the Decipher in recent time is considered the most powerful method in that it comprises of a comprehensive transcriptome investigation of a prostatectomy, biopsy, or transurethral resection specimens. Interestingly, the Decipher method for evaluation of PCa prognostication was initially authenticated in radical prostatectomy patients with uncomplimentary specimen characteristics inclusive of positive cancer margins and is however independent of clinical data [33–35, 107]. A study by Den et al. found that the Decipher method demonstrated both biochemical recurrence and cancer spreading in approximate 139 participants after removal of the prostate in addition to radiotherapy [36].

Several authors have done in-depth assessment and evaluation of the clinical utility of the Decipher method in PCa progression. Spratt et al. performed a meta-analysis of 5 studies comprising 855 patients in assessing the performance of the Decipher test in PCa patients who underwent radical post-prostatectomy. The Decipher test classified patients as low, intermediate and high risk for developing metastases and was a significant predictor of metastasis (HR = 1.30, p < 0.001). The authors posited that the Decipher test can increase the prognosis of PCa patients after radical prostatectomy including those in the different clinicopathologic and therapy subgroups (**Table 1**) [33]. Similarly, the prognostic potential of the Decipher test was assessed in two high-risk USA and European case-control studies. The median Decipher scores were higher in PCa patients who developed metastases, and multivariate analysis showed that there was a greater risk of distant metastases for each 10% increase in Decipher score within a 10-year follow-up period. Therefore, the Decipher test predicted metastatic recurrence in PCa patients within a follow-up period of 10 years [37]. In a retrospective multicenter cohort study comprising of 266 PCa patients, the Decipher from prostatectomies from PCa patients with low to intermediate risk predicted the absence of adverse pathologic features thus making these individuals suitable for active surveillance [38]. In a later study involving prostatectomies from 2342 PCa patients, the Decipher score was positively correlated with baseline tumor characteristics such as age, pathologic T-stage and GS [39]. The Decipher score was able to reclassify patients according to tumor aggressiveness and may be valuable in assessing postoperative risk and decision making [39].

There are other studies that have assessed the clinical usefulness of the Decipher test in risk stratification of newly diagnosed PCa patients. In a multicenter prospective study involving 855 persons who underwent Decipher Biopsy testing, a high-risk Decipher score for PCa patients in the active surveillance group was independently associated with time to treatment while the same was related to time to failure in the radical therapy group [40]. Likewise, in a study of 203 PCa cases, the Decipher score enables risk stratification and was significantly associated with time to biochemical recurrence. The Decipher score could assist PCa patients with treatment decision as high-risk values were significantly associated with salvage treatment [40]. Interestingly, a systematic review conducted recently of 42 studies and 3407 patients [localized, post-prostatectomy, metastatic castration resistant PCa (mCRPCa) and metastatic hormone sensitive PCa (mHSPCa)], and metastatic hormone sensitive PCa (mHSPCa), the Decipher test was robust for intermediate-risk PCa and decision-making after radical prostatectomy [41].

The Decipher test has been used in risk stratification of early diagnosed PCa patients and for treatment making decisions [108]. Dalela et al. investigated the use of the Decipher test in a cohort of 512 PCa patients as a valuable risk-stratification tool for identifying those persons who would be received maximum benefit from adjuvant radiotherapy (ART). The Decipher test was one of the parameters used to develop a Multivariable Prediction Model that predicted reduced risk for clinical recurrence. Using the Decipher test, the authors suggested that ART might decrease overtreatment and needless adverse effects [34]. Also, supporting evidence was observed in the Multicenter Prospective PRO-IMPACT study comprising of 150 PCa patients where the Decipher score acts as a guide for making treatment choice, and enhance the effectiveness of the decision-making process for PCa patients considering salvage radiotherapy (SRT) or ART post-radical prostatectomy [35]. The use of the Decipher test has been found to significantly improve therapy decision-making in a study published of two prospective registries of PCa patients [42]. Of particular interest is a study by Lobo et al. which based on the findings suggests that the Decipher test was a cost-effective approach to PCa treatment decisions after radical prostatectomy. This should result in improved clinical outcomes and the potential for the application of the Decipher test for personalized cancer medicine [109].

3.3.3 ConfirmMDx

ConfirmDx is a tissue based biomarker that is used to determine the likelihood of a true negative biopsy versus one that has an occult cancer. The aim of this test is to prevent unnecessary repeat biopsies and also to detect those patients with negative biopsies who in fact, do require repeat biopsies. Unnecessary biopsies put patients at risk for complications from the biopsy procedure and increases morbidity, in addition to increasing economic burden.

Prostate biopsies are done when there is an increase in tPSA level and/or abnormal prostate DRE. When a prostate biopsy is negative and there is a high suspicion of

PCa, the residual tissue from the biopsy can be submitted for the ConfirmMDx test. ConfirmMDx is an epigenetic assay that is used to detect DNA hyper-methylation changes. Epigenetic changes such as DNA methylation have been implicated in the molecular pathogenesis of PCa. These changes occur surrounding the tumor foci, called the halo effect. It occurs within a DNA sequence, when a methyl group is added to a cytosine nucleotide that is adjacent to a guanine nucleotide [110]. The three genes tested for DNA hyper-methylation associated with PCa are: GSTP1, APC, and RASSF1 genes [110]. Unlike histopathology of a prostate core biopsy which would have missed the diagnosis of epigenetic changes, these 3 genes have the potential to expose the presence of tumor activity via the use of ConfirmMDx.

From the methylation analysis to locate occult cancer (MATLOC) study conducted in 2013, the rate of false negative results from prostate biopsies was significantly lowered with a 90% NPV when compared with histopathology. Specificity and sensitivity were found to be 64% and 68% respectively [111]. Moreover, another study to substantiate the MATLOC study was the DOCUMENT (detection of cancer using methylated events in negative tissue) trial done in 2013. This resulted in a NPV of 88% (95% Cl 85–91) [49]. This was significant for repeat biopsies as an independent predictor of PCa.

In another study, Waterhouse et al. in 2018 found that ConfirmMDx used for PCa detection had a sensitivity and specificity of 74.1% and 60.0% respectively at repeat biopsies. The study validated the use of ConfirmMDx in African American men, and was significant as most studies were done on a Caucasian population [50]. Further, Wojno et al., found that PCa patients who were managed using ConfirmMDx test had a <5% rate of repeat prostate biopsies. Compared with previous rates, there was a tenfold reduction [51]. ConfirmMDx test has the potential therefore, to reduce healthcare costs by avoiding unnecessary repeat biopsies and to also avoid the morbidity associated with prostate biopsies. Notably, ConfirmMDx is not FDA approved.

3.4 Emerging molecular prostate cancer biomarkers

3.4.1 The ProMark

There are challenges in defining the aggressiveness of PCa as well as its outcome (particularly lethality) using prostate biopsy as there are sample errors and disparities in interpretation. Shipitsin et al. documented a proteomic biopsy-based PCa prognostic advanced test panel called ProMark that is manufactured and distributed by Metamark Genetics Incorporated, USA. They performed and documented a result-orientated method that provides an accurate prognosis of PCa aggressiveness and lethal outcome irrespective of variation in biopsy sampling [112]. Using a large patient cohort, prostatectomy tissue samples were identified and classified as having lowest to the highest Gleason grade. Tissue microarrays were produced comprising of cores from low as well as high Gleason area from each PCa patient. An assessment of 160 known protein biomarkers was carried out by means of using a quantitative multiplex proteomics in situ imaging system and a selection strategy with three types of criteria namely biological, technical and performance-based. Analytical performance and the application of univariate and multivariate analyses resulted in a final set of 12 protein biomarkers which provided prognostic accuracy of tumor behavior [113]. The same researchers conducted further investigations with the subsequent selection of 8 of these 12 protein biomarkers in a prognostic model that offered "risk scores" predictive of the final post-prostatectomy pathology.

The eight proteomic biomarkers that constitute ProMark are: HSPA9, YBX1, CUL2, PDSS2, pS6, FUS, DERL1 and SMAD4 [52].

Blume-Jensen et al. performed a multicenter 8-protein biomarker assay model investigation involving 381 PCa patient biopsies with corresponding prostatectomy specimens. This was followed by a second blinded study of 276 cases which validated the 8-protein biomarker assay model's capacity to differentiate "non-favorable" versus "favorable" pathology in a manner that was independent and comparative to D'Amico and National Comprehensive Cancer Network (NCCN). The protein biomarker panel of ProMark gives a risk score ranging from 0 to 1 and predicts the aggressiveness of PCa and lethal outcome in patients with GS of 3 + 4 and 3 + 3 on biopsy. There was a false positive rate of 5% that corresponds to a non-favorable protein biomarker assay risk score >0.80 and false negative rate of 10% which relates to favorable protein biomarker assay risk score <0.33 [52]. The ProMark predictive model gave values for favorable pathology (risk score ≤ 0.33) of 87.2% for patients in the low-risk D'Amico group, as well as 81.5% and 95.0% for those in the low-risk and very low-risk NCCN groups respectively. These predictive values were higher than those of the up-to-date risk classification groups (70.6%—low-risk D'Amico group; 63.8%—low-risk NCCN; 80.3%—very low-risk NCCN respectively). The ProMark predictive model gave a value for non-favorable pathology (risk score > 0.80) of 76.9% for all the NCCN and D'Amico risk groups. The validation study of the 8-protein biomarker assay predictive model was able to distinguish non-favorable from favorable (AUC = 0.68; p < 0.0001; OR = 20.9) and GS 3 + 3 versus GS 3 + 4 (AUC = 0.65; p < 0.0001; OR = 12.95) [52]. Overall, with increasing ProMark biomarker risk scores there was reduced frequency of favorable PCa cases across all the D'Amico and NCCN risk groups [52].

3.4.2 miRNAs

3.4.2.1 Diagnosis, progression, risk stratification and therapeutic potential of serum or plasma miRNAs

MicroRNAs (miRNAs) are minute single-stranded as well as non-coding sections in RNA comprising of approximately 22 nucleotides that pay a critical role in gene regulation [53]. In the past decade a number of studies have investigated the differential expression and levels of miRNAs in plasma or serum in order to develop non-invasive blood-based biomarkers with the ability to diagnose, detect progression and assess prognosis as well as recurrence of PCa [114]. Jin et al. investigated 10 serum-circulating miRNAs as non-invasive molecular biomarkers in 31 BPH and 31 PCa patients. The expression levels of miR-375, miR-200b, and miR-141 levels were significantly elevated in the PCa patients compared with those in the BPH group, and miR-200b was the most effective diagnostic marker with AUC = 0.923 [115]. An association was found between the three miRNAs and tPSA, as well as miR-200b and GS [115]. The upregula-tion of miR-141 was also observed in a study by Ibrahim et al. that comprised 80 PCa (30 metastatic and 50 localized), 30 BPH patients and 50 healthy controls (**Table 2**). Plasma miR-141, miR-221, miR-18a and miR-21 levels were significantly higher in PCa patients than healthy controls. miR-18a differentiate PCa from healthy individuals with the highest AUC of 0.966, while miR-221 has a sensitivity of 92.9% and specificity of 100% at differentiating localized from metastatic PCa [116]. Likewise, another study differentiated PCa from BPH as higher significant expressions of the two onco-mRNAs miR-375-3p and miR-182-5p were found in the plasma of PCa compared with BPH patients (specificity = 90.2%) [131]. Similarly, the expressions levels of miR-375-3p

miRNA Identified	Study type	Specimen	Outcome	References
miR-141, miR-182, miR-200b, and miR-375	31 PCa and BPH patients	Serum	Diagnosis	[115]
miR-21, miR-141, miR-18a and miR-221	80 PCa, 30 BPH and 50 controls	Plasma	Diagnosis	[116]
miR-494	90 PCa and 90 BPH	Serum	Diagnosis	[117]
miR-301a	13 BPH and 28 PCa	Serum and tissue	Diagnosis/ prognosis	[118]
miR-410-5p	149 PCa, 121BPH and 57 controls	Serum	Diagnosis	[119]
miR-320a/-b/-c	145 PCa, 31 BPH and 19 controls	Serum	Diagnosis	[120]
miR-128	129 PCa patients	Serum and tissue	Diagnosis, prognosis	[121]
miR-628-5p	40 PCa patients and 32 controls	Serum	Diagnosis, prognosis	[122]
miR-4286, miR-27a-3p, and miR-29b-3p	78 PCa and 77 BPH	Serum	Diagnosis	[123]
miR-15a, miR-126, miR-192 and miR-377	35 PCa, 35 BPH and 30 controls	Serum	Diagnosis/risk	[124]
let-7b, miR-34a, miR-125b, miR-143, miR-miR-145 and miR-221	2 Prospective cohorts (12 mPCa and 25 controls; 149 PCa patients)	Plasma and tissue	Diagnosis	[125]
miR-210-3p, miR-23c, miR-592 and miR-93-5p	159 PCa fresh tissues and 60 plasma samples	Plasma and tissue	Risk stratification	[126]
miR-141-3p and miR-375-3p	84 mCRPCa patients	Serum	Therapy	[127]
miR-1825, miR-484, miR-205, miR-141, and let-7b	72 PCa and 34 controls	Serum	Prognosis/ therapy	[128]
miRNA-223, miRNA-24 and miRNA-375	196 PCa patients for training and 133 PCa patients for validation	Serum	Surveillance	[129]
miR-200c and miR-200b	102 PCa patients and 50 controls	Plasma	Diagnosis, prognosis	[130]

Table 2.
Summary of miRNA expression studies on plasma or serum samples from prostate cancer patients.

and miR-182-5p were evaluated for their diagnostic and prognostic potential in a cohort of 98 PCa and 52 normal controls. The plasma miR-182-5p expression level was significantly higher in PCa patients compared with controls, and it detected the disease with AUC = 0.64 (specificity of 77% and NPV of 99%). The authors also found that the levels of both miRNAs were associated with higher GS, and miR-182-5p was significantly elevated in metastatic PCa [132].

miRNAs exhibited both diagnostic and prognostic ability and these could be considered for possible use in clinical practice [108]. Cai and Peng investigated the diagnostic potential of miR-494 in a study comprising 90 BPH and 90 PCa patients, and 90 healthy controls. The serum expression of miR-494 was significantly higher in PCa compared with BPH patients and healthy controls, and positively correlated with GS, tumor size and stage, and serum tPSA levels. miR-494 was suggested to be a sensitive biomarker of PCa as the AUC was 0.809 [117]. A similar investigation was carried out for miR-301a extracted from serum and tumor samples in a study design involving two cohorts (cohort 1 of 13 BPH and 25 PCa, and cohort 2 of 12 BPH and 13PCa). miRNA-301a expression in serum and tissue was significantly higher in PCa compared with BPH patients, and there was correlation with increased GS for miR-301a in radical prostatectomy specimens [118]. Also, miR-410-5p was investigated as a potential serum biomarker for PCa in a study comprising 149 PCa and 121 BPH patients, and 57 healthy controls. The serum expression of miR-410-5p was significantly elevated in PCa compared with BPH patients or healthy controls. The diagnostic accuracy of serum miR-410-5p indicated by an AUC of 0.810 suggests that it is a potential molecular biomarker for the diagnosis of PCa [119].

Other miRNAs have been overexpressed or under-expressed in circulation thus demonstrating their diagnostic and prognostic potentials. Lieb et al. in a study of 145 PCa and BPH patients, and 19 healthy controls reported that the serum levels of miRNA family members (miR-320a, miR-320b and miR-320c) differed among the three groups been highest in the PCa patients. In addition, the serum levels of all three miRNAs were significantly higher in older patients, high tumor stage and those with tPSA >4 ng/mL [120]. Conversely, decreased miR-128 expression was found in the serum of 128 PCa patients which was associated with disease progression and short biochemical recurrence-free survival (**Table 2**) [121].

miRNA profiling experiments followed by validation showed decreased expression of serum miR-25, miR-628-5p, and miR-101 in African American and Caucasian Americans with PCa compared with healthy controls [122]. Other serum or plasma miRNAs which have been identified as potential non-invasive biomarkers for PCa include: has-miR-101-3p and has-miR-19b-39 (diagnosis and prognosis) [133], miR-940 (diagnosis, AUC = 0.75) [134], panel of miR-27a-3p, miR-424-5p, miR-29b-3p, miR-4286 and miR-365a-3p (detecting early stage PCa) [123], panel of miR-126, miR-377, miR-15a and miR-192 (detection of localized PCa and risk stratification) [124] as well as panel of miR-373, miR-141, miR-21, miR-125b, miR-126, miR143 and let-7b (diagnosis of metastatic PCa) (**Table 2**) [125].

3.4.2.2 Diagnosis, prognosis and therapeutic potential of miRNAs in tissue

The profiling of miRNAs in tissues of PCa patients shows pattern that are different compared with those from healthy controls. These distinct miRNA expressions in PCa tissues could afford tools for improved diagnosis, prognosis and therapeutic approaches for PCa [114]. Huang et al. investigated the clinical utility and prognostic potential of hsa-miR-30c and hsa-miR-203 in tissues of 44 PCa patients. The expressions of the two miRNAs in tumor tissues were significantly different from those in neighboring normal tissue indicating their diagnostic potential. All the PCa patients were followed up for 36 months and the data showed that the mean survival times of high and low expressions of hsa-miR-203 and has-miR-30c respectively were significantly lower, which attest to their possible prognostic utility for PCa [135]. In a study involving tissue samples from 14 BPH and 60 PCa patients (cancerous and noncancerous prostate samples) and the employment of qRT-PCR followed by validation, the expression levels of 4 miRNAs (miRNA-141-5p, miR-183-5p, miR-32-5p and 187-3p) differed significantly between PCa and BPH samples [136]. The data suggests that these four miRNAs could detect cancer in prostate biopsy as they were able to differentiate between malignant and nonmalignant prostates [136]. Likewise, the expressions of miR-27b were higher in PCa compared with BPH tissues, and correlated with GS and clinical stages in PCa. The researchers further posited that PCa patients with higher expression of miR-27b had worse progression free as well as overall survival [137]. There are other studies that have shown an overexpression of miR-153 in PCa tissue which was associated with worse overall survival (**Table 3**) [145], and the deregulation of miR-30c and miR-29b with decreased expression in PCa tissues and ability to differentiate between PCa and adjacent para-cancerous tissues (AUC = 0.944 for miR-30c and AUC = 0.924 for miR-29b) (**Table 3**) [138].

There are a few studies that have investigated the therapeutic potential of miRNAs for PCa treatment because of their ability to bind targets using prostate tissue and cell lines [149]. Wang et al. explored the prognostic potential and possible use of miR-1231 as a therapeutic tool by measuring its expression levels in PCa tissues. The miR-1231 expression was decreased in PCa tissues and significantly associated with shorter overall survival, higher TNM stage, lymph node metastasis and higher clinical stage. The data also showed that epidermal growth factor receptor (EGFR) is a target

miRNA Identified	Study type	Specimen	Outcome	References
miR-128	128 PCa cases	Tissue	Prognosis	[121]
hsa-miR-203 and hsa-miR-30c	44 PCa patients	Tissue	Diagnosis, prognosis	[135]
miR-187-3p, miR-183-5p, miR-32-5p, and miR-141-5p	14 BPH and 60 PCa tissue samples	Tissue	Diagnostics	[136]
miR-30c and miR-29b	187 cases of PCa	Tissue	Diagnosis	[138]
miR-424-3p	Prostatectomy specimens 535 PCa patients	Tissue	Therapy	[139]
miR-20b	127 PCa patients	Tissue	Prognosis	[140]
miR-17-5p	535 PCa patients	Tissue	Prognosis	[141]
miR-148b-3p	PCa and BPH samples	Tissue	Diagnosis	[142]
miR-1231	PCa tissues and cell lines	Tissue	Prognostic, therapy	[143]
miR-615-3p	239 PCa patients	Tissue	Prognosis	[144]
miR-153	143 pairs of PCa tissues	Tissue	Prognosis	[145]
miR-130b	PCa tissue from African Americans	Tissue	Prognosis and race disparity	[146]
miR-27b	28 BPH and 63 PCa tissues	Tissue	Diagnosis, prognosis	[137]
miR-1207-3p	404 post-prostatectomy prostate tumor tissue samples	Tissue	Prognosis	[147]
miR-301a	75 formalin fixed paraffin embedded localized PCa tissue, 4 mPCa tissue and 13 BPH tissue	Tissue	Prognosis	[148]

Table 3.
Summary of miRNA expression studies on tissue from prostate cancer patients.

of miR-1231 and its over-expression reduced migration, proliferation and invasion of PCa cell lines in vitro. Based on the evidence, the researchers suggested that miR-1231 has a tumor-suppressive role, may be a prognostic biomarker, and a therapeutic tool for PCa treatment in the future (**Table 3**) [143]. In another study involving naïve radical prostatectomy specimens from 535 PCa patients, decreased expression of miR-424-3p was significantly associated with the aggressive phenotype of PCa and clinical failure-free survival. Based on the evidence, the authors posited that miR-424-3p could be a possible target for treatment of PCa (**Table 3**) [139].

3.4.3 Exosomes

Exosomes are minute membrane-bound extracellular vesicles with diameters of 30–150 nm. They are released from many cell types into body fluids and the extracellular environs after the amalgamation of multi-vesicular bodies fuse with the plasma membrane [150]. Exosomes comprised of a number of cytoplasmic biomolecules such as lipids, glycol-conjugates, proteins, DNA and RNA including miRNAs surrounded by a lipid bilayer membrane. They are found in blood (plasma and serum), urine, saliva and semen and cell culture medium [140, 151]. During PCa development and metastasis, exosomes are secreted by tumor cells and have been reported to play a critical role in initiation, promotion, immuno-regulation, angiogenesis, annexation and metastasis [152]. As exosomes play a role in PCa development via a number of mechanisms of actions, they are valuable biomarkers for PCa diagnosis, prognosis and monitoring [153, 154].

3.4.3.1 Exosome-contained microRNAs

Exosomal miRNAs are small-stranded non-coding RNA (about 17–25 nucleotides in length) and changes in their concentration in body fluids make them useful molecular biomarkers of PCa progression [155]. There is increasing interest in exosomal miRNAs in serum and plasma samples due to their stability and as non-invasive molecular biomarkers for PCa diagnosis and recurrence [156]. Li et al. conducted a study comprising 31 PCa patients and 19 healthy persons and found that plasma exosomal miR-125a-5p levels were significantly decreased in the former compared with the latter. The researchers also found that plasma exosomal miR-141-5p levels mildly increased in PCa patients, and the miR-125a-5p/miR-141-5p ratio was able to distinguish these patients from healthy controls (AUC = 0.793) [157].

In a recent study, Guo et al. examined the predictive potential of 6 plasma exosomal miRNAs in a first validation prospective cohort of 42 CRPCa and 108 treatment-naive PCa patients, and found that miR-423-3p was associated with CRPCa (AUC = 0.784). In a second validation study reported by the same authors, plasma exosomal miR-423-3p expression was significantly higher in 30 CRPCa patients undergoing androgen depletion treatment compared with 36 non-CRPCa patients (AUC = 0.879). The authors suggested that plasma exosomal miR-423-3p may serve as a useful molecular biomarker for early diagnosis and prognosis of castration resistance in PCa patients [153]. Moreover, in an earlier study that examined the overall survival in a prospective cohort of 23 CRPCa patients, significantly elevated levels of plasma exosomal miR-375 and miR-1290 were associated with worse clinical outcome and overall survival in CRPCa patients [158].

There are serum exosomal miRNAs that are investigated for potential clinical utility for PCa. In an investigation by Li et al., the expression of serum exosomal miR-141 was significantly higher in PCa patients compared with those of BPH patients and healthy individuals. Serum exosomal miR-141 expression was also significantly higher in PCa patients with metastasis compared with localized disease. The authors suggested that serum exosomal miR-141 could be a valuable molecular biomarker for the diagnosis of metastatic PCa [159]. In preclinical vivo and in vitro studies, exosomal miR-1246, a tumor suppressor was downregulated in PCa cell lines, and clinical tissues correlated with the presence of metastasis, poor prognosis and increasing GS [160].

Urinary exosomal miRNAs have been found to be valuable noninvasive and diagnostic molecular biomarkers of PCa [161]. Shin et al. investigated the clinical utility and profiles of urinary exosomal miRNA expressions in 149 PCa cases and the identification of those associated with metastasis. Urinary exosomal miR-21 and miR-451 expressions were upregulated and miR-636 downregulated in metastatic PCa patients compared to those with localized disease. These three exosomal miRNAs were used to develop a Prostate Cancer Metastasis Risk Scoring (PCa-MRS) model for PCa patients with high scores showing significantly worse biochemical recurrence-free survival [162]. Similarly, in a recent study comprising of a next-generation sequencing cohort (6 PCa patients and 3 healthy individuals) and use of qRT-PCR (28 BPH patients, 47 PCa patients and 25 gender- and age-matched healthy controls), urinary exosomal miR-486-5p, miR-486-3p, miR-375, miR-486-5p and miR-451a expressions discriminated PCa patients from healthy controls with AUCs ranging from 0.704 to 0.796. The researchers found that urinary exosomal miR-375 differentiated metastatic PCa from localized (AUC = 0.806), and miR-451a along with miR-375 distinguished localized PCa from BPH (AUC = 0.726) [155]. In an earlier study comprising 90 PCa patients, 10 BPH and 50 healthy controls, urinary exosomal miR-2909 was reported to be a non-invasive diagnostic molecular biomarker of PCa and disease aggressiveness [163]. Preclinical studies also revealed that urinary exosomal miR-574-3p and miR-375 were detected by molecular beacons in PCa cells such as PC-3 and DU145 [164]. Furthermore, urinary exosomal miR-532-5p expression was upregulated in 26 PCa patients with biochemical recurrence and exhibit poor prognosis in those with intermediate-risk disease [165].

The findings from these observational studies indicated that circulating exosomal miRNAs in serum, plasma or urine may assist in the diagnosis, prognosis and outcomes of PCa and could be adopted into routine clinical practice in the near future.

3.5 Potential prostate cancer biomarkers in development

3.5.1 Prostarix

Prostarix is another PCa biomarker that has potential value in screening/diagnosis. It is a post-DRE urine test that is used to predict the likelihood of having a negative prostate biopsy versus one with occult PCa. This is done using a risk score. The risk score is generated using an algorithm which ranges from 0% to 100%. One hundred percent equates to a 100% chance of having PCa on a prostate biopsy. Therefore, it is used to determine which men will undergo prostate biopsy. Prostarix is used when there is an elevated tPSA and normal DRE, and in some cases, for men who are candidates for a repeat prostate biopsy [166, 167].

Prostarix measures four metabolites using liquid chromatography mass spectrometry. These metabolites are sarcosine, alanine, glycine and glutamate. Sarcosine especially, has been linked with PCa progression [168]. A study conducted by McDunn et al. 2013, showed that these metabolites improved prediction of organ confinement (AUC, 0.53–0.62) and 5-year recurrence (AUC, 0.53–0.64) [166]. However, a study done by Sroka et al. in 2017 that evaluated various amino acids as PCa biomarkers found that sarcosine was not a definitive indicator of PCa when analyzed in pre and post-prostate massage urine samples. Also, the amino acids arginine, homoserine, and proline were mostly seen in the urine samples of PCa patients as opposed to patients with a benign prostatic disease [169]. It is evident that more studies need to be done on Prostarix, and of note, it is not FDA approved.

3.5.2 Prostate Core Mitomic Test

Prostate Core Mitomic Test (PCMT) is a tissue based biomarker for detecting PCa. It is an RT-PCR test that detects large-scale mitochondrial deletions in prostate biopsy samples. It is able to identify tumor activity at the molecular level and detects molecular changes that occur at the mitochondrial DNA (mDNA) level. The large-scale deletion of 3.4 kb of the mitochondrial genome has been known to occur as a part of the prostate "cancerization" field effect [170]. Cancerization field effect occurs when cells adjacent to primary tumors become transformed [171]. This takes place at the start of oncogenesis. Cancerization field effect is seen in some type of cancers including PCa. Histopathology would have otherwise labeled these prostate biopsy samples with cancerization field effects as "normal" appearing tissue.

PCMT is used to predict repeat biopsy outcomes with an initial negative biopsy. This test can therefore, aid in reduction of the number of unnecessary biopsies and also reduce health care costs. According to Robinson et al. in 2010, the sensitivity and specificity of this mitochondrial deletion in predicting repeat biopsy outcomes were found to be 84% and 54% respectively. It also showed a NPV of 91% and an AUC of 0.749 [172]. Legisi et al. performed a multicenter observational study to assess the use of the PCMT in the decision making of repeated biopsy among patients with a strong suspicion of PCa. Using two independent query language databases, the PCMT addressed sampling errors related to prostate biopsy and gave more evidence concerning the clinical uncertainty surrounding an initial negative prostate biopsy [173]. Notably, the PCMT is not FDA approved.

4. Discussion

Globally, PCa is regarded as the most predominant malignancy in males and the principal cause of cancer-related mortality. Given the negative impact of PCa as it relates to morbidity and quality of life as well as mortality, early detection of the disease is of critical importance. Presently, tPSA and DRE are used in the diagnosis of PCa but there are a number of limitations which include low specificity and sensitivity leading to over-diagnosis and subsequent unnecessary prostate biopsies. In the early stage of PCa development there are no symptoms so there is a need for biochemical and molecular diagnostic tests for accurate and prompt detection. This review documents a number of PCa diagnostic and prognostics tests that have been discovered in the last two decades due to improvements in genomic technologies. Among them are serum PHI and 4K score, urine PCA3 and SelectMDx, and tumor tissue Oncotype DX, Decipher and Prolarix. These biomarkers are used in clinical decision making for PCa such as suspected patients who are required to undertake an initial prostate biopsy, or those who need a second biopsy given that the initial one was negative for the disease. These tests have generated new prospects for advancing PCa diagnosis, prognosis such as the prediction of metastatic disease recurrence and decisions regarding therapy. In particular, Oncotype DX afford information regarding risk stratification which aid in identifying PCa patients that should receive treatment after a positive prostate biopsy, and Decipher those individuals to be treated post-surgery [174].

There have been a substantial number of miRNA-based assays and evidence in the literature demonstrates increased or decreased expression levels of miRNAs in peripheral blood (serum and plasma), prostate tissues and body fluids (urine and seminal) that differentiate between PCa and BPH patients, as well as healthy controls. This review presented findings on the clinical utility of miRNAs as diagnostic and prognostic biomarkers, and possible therapeutic targets for PCa. The findings are encouraging particularly the downregulation or upregulation of miRNAs expressions in plasma, serum or urine which facilitates the non-invasive nature, fast and cost-effectiveness of the tests. However, significant work is warranted if the miRNAs biomarkers are to translate from bench to routine clinical use. Also, larger observational prospective studies are needed with the intent of substantiating the validity of miRNAs and determining precise stratification based on the expression levels of miRNAs in PCa at different stages along the continuum of the disease. Furthermore, there are issues to be addressed such as the absence of guidelines for miRNAs development including isolation protocols, differences in study designs, pre-analytical variables such as specimen collection issues and tumor heterogeneity, need for validation and the selection of the best detection method (qRT-PCR vs. microarray) [175].

The presence of proteins and miRNAs in exosomes of prostate tissues makes them a valuable molecular diagnostic biomarker and therapeutic tool for PCa treatment. The development of these biomarkers is still in its early stages, but the results are very encouraging. The evidence presented in this review suggests that serum, plasma and urine exosomal miRNAs are useful for early detection as it differentiate metastatic from localized PCa together with prognosis of mCRPCa. There is a paucity of studies on exosomal proteins such as serum claudin 3 and survivin as well as urine-based LAMTOR1, TMEM256 and PARK7. This is an exciting area and research is continuing. However, there are challenges such as the complex process of obtaining appropriate samples, the lack of suitable isolation protocols and the need to standardized purification and quantification methods [176]. Overcoming these obstacles in preclinical research could result in these exosomal biomarkers being applied in the clinical setting for risk stratification, prognosis and the monitoring of PCa.

Moreover, PCa biomarkers employ diverse types of samples such as blood (serum or plasma), urine, prostate tissue (specimen from transurethral resection, biopsy and radical prostatectomy) and seminal fluid [177]. Assays comprising these PCa biomarkers are evaluated as their clinical use involved improving early diagnosis and risk stratification of localized tumor, reducing the number of needless biopsies with subsequent saving on use of expensive intervention strategies [177].

Traditionally blood, a minimally invasive and easily obtained sample is the chief source of PCa biomarkers for example serum tPSA and in recent years emerging biomarkers such miRNA has been developed. Panels for new PCa biomarkers will permit fingerprinting of the biologic behavior of the tumor with possibly personalized therapy and monitoring [178]. The collection of urine sample for the assessment of PCa biomarkers is a simple, non-invasive approach and assays can be used to monitor PCa with heterogeneous tumor foci [179]. Currently some of the emerging protein and non-protein non-invasive urinary PCa biomarkers comprise TMPRSS2, PCA3, miRNAs and SelectMDx [180]. Genomic studies and biotechnological advancement have improved the sensitivity and specificity of these urinary PCa biomarkers thus enhanced clinical outcomes relating to early diagnosis and better selection of treatment approaches [181].

Tissue-based PCa biomarkers are invasive and fewer, and in the area of molecular diagnostics there is more focus on assays for blood and urine-based biomarkers with diagnostic and prognostic potential. However, there is growing interest on tissue-based PCa biomarkers such as ProMark, Oncotype DX and Decipher as well as miRNA and exosomal miRNA [182].

Finally, there are emerging molecular biomarkers that are at different phases of development, and many are in the preclinical phase. It is hope that in the next decade or so a significant collection of biomarkers with excellent diagnostic good sensitivity and specificity together with significant prognostic potential will be available for use by physicians in the clinical setting [183–185].

5. Conclusion

This review provides evidence of the use of established and emerging biomarkers detected in body fluids as diagnostic and prognostic tools for PCa. Despite the promising findings in preclinical and clinical research among the increasing body of investigations, there are challenges which delay the translation of a number of biomarkers from bench to bedside. Nonetheless, the considerable prospect of the biomarkers such as miRNAs and exosomal miRNAs in clinical practice as therapeutic tools for PCa is widely acknowledged and hopefully will be a reality in the not too distant future.

Nothing to disclose

The authors have no funding and conflicts of interest to disclose regarding the content of this chapter.

Author details

Donovan McGrowder[1*], Lennox Anderson-Jackson[1], Lowell Dilworth[1],
Shada Mohansingh[1], Melisa Anderson Cross[2], Sophia Bryan[3], Fabian Miller[4,5],
Cameil Wilson-Clarke[3], Chukwuemeka Nwokocha[3], Ruby Alexander-Lindo[3]
and Shelly McFarlane[6]

1 Faculty of Medical Sciences, Department of Pathology, The University of the West
Indies, Kingston, Jamaica

2 School of Allied Health and Wellness, College of Health Sciences, University of
Technology, Kingston, Jamaica

3 Faculty of Medical Sciences, Department of Basic Medical Sciences, The University
of the West Indies, Kingston, Jamaica

4 Faculty of Science and Technology, Department of Biotechnology, The University of
the West Indies, Kingston, Jamaica

5 Faculty of Education, Department of Physical Education, The Mico University
College, Kingston, Jamaica

6 Faculty of Medical Sciences, Caribbean Institute for Health Research, The
University of the West Indies, Kingston, Jamaica

*Address all correspondence to: dmcgrowd@yahoo.com

IntechOpen

References

[1] Sung H, Ferlay J, Siegel RL, Laversanne M, Soerjomataram I, Jemal A, et al. Global cancer statistics 2020: GLOBOCAN estimates of incidence and mortality worldwide for 36 cancers in 185 countries. CA: A Cancer Journal for Clinicians. 2021;**71**(3):209-249

[2] Siegel RL, Miller KD, Jemal A. Cancer statistics, 2020. CA: A Cancer Journal for Clinicians. 2020;**70**(1):7-30

[3] Siegel R, Ma J, Zou Z, Jemal A. Cancer statistics, 2014. CA: A Cancer Journal for Clinicians. 2014;**64**(1):9-29

[4] Cuzick J, Thorat MA, Andriole G, Brawley OW, Brown PH, Culig Z, et al. Prevention and early detection of prostate cancer. Lancet Oncology. 2014;**15**(11):e484-e492

[5] DeSantis CE, Siegel RL, Sauer AG, Miller KD, Fedewa SA, Alcaraz KI, et al. Cancer statistics for African Americans, 2016: Progress and opportunities in reducing racial disparities. CA: A Cancer Journal for Clinicians. 2016;**66**(4):290-308

[6] Fornara P, Theil G, Schaefer C, Heß J, Rübben H. Benefits and risks of prostate cancer screening. Oncology Research and Treatment. 2014;**37**(suppl 3):29-37

[7] Parekh DJ, Punnen S, Sjoberg DD, Asroff SW, Bailen JL, Cochran JW, et al. A multi-institutional prospective trial in the USA confirms that the 4Kscore accurately identifies men with high-grade prostate cancer. European Urology. 2015;**68**(3):464-470

[8] Tokudome S, Ando R, Koda Y. Discoveries and application of prostate specific antigen, and some proposals to optimize prostate cancer screening. Cancer Management and Research. 2016;**8**:45-47

[9] Roddam AW, Duffy MJ, Hamdy FC, et al. Use of prostate-specific antigen (PSA) isoforms for the detection of prostate cancer in men with a PSA level of 2-10 ng/ml: Systematic review and meta-analysis. European Urology. 2005;**48**:386-399

[10] Shariat SF, Scardino PT, Lilja H. Screening for prostate cancer: An update. The Canadian Journal of Urology. 2008;**15**(6):4363-4374

[11] Filella X, Fernández-Galan E, Fernández Bonifacio R, Foj L. Emerging biomarkers in the diagnosis of prostate cancer. Pharmacogenomics and Personalized Medicine. 2018;**11**:83-94

[12] Carneiro A, Priante Kayano P, Gomes Barbosa ÁR, Langer Wroclawski M, Ko Chen C, Cavlini GC, et al. Are localized prostate cancer biomarkers useful in the clinical practice? Tumour Biology. 2018;**40**(9):1010428318799255. DOI: 10.1177/1010428318799255

[13] Mao Z, Ji A, Yang K, He W, Hu Y, Zhang Q, et al. Diagnostic performance of PCA3 and hK2 in combination with serum PSA for prostate cancer. Medicine (Baltimore). 2018;**97**(42):e12806. DOI: 10.1097/MD.0000000000012806

[14] Saini S. PSA and beyond: Alternative prostate cancer biomarkers. Cellular Oncology (Dordrecht). 2016;**39**(2):97-106

[15] Porzycki P, Ciszkowicz E. Modern biomarkers in prostate cancer diagnosis. Central European Journal of Urology. 2020;**73**(3):300-306

[16] Thompson IM, Ankerst DP, Chi C, Lucia MS, Goodman PJ, Crowley JJ, et al. Operating characteristics of prostate-specific antigen in men with an initial PSA level of 3.0 ng/mL or lower. Journal of the American Medical Association. 2005;**294**(1):66-70

[17] Hayes JH, Barry MJ. Screening for prostate cancer with the prostate - specific antigen test: A review of current evidence. Journal of the American Medical Association. 2014;**311**:1143-1149

[18] Liu J, Dong B, Qu W, Wang J, Xu Y, Yu S, et al. Using clinical parameters to predict prostate cancer and reduce the unnecessary biopsy among patients with PSA in the gray zone. Scientific Reports. 2020;**10**(1):5157. DOI: 10.1038/s41598-020-62015-w

[19] Mikolajczyk SD, Rittenhouse HG. Tumor-associated forms of prostate specific antigen improve the discrimination of prostate cancer from benign disease. Rinsho Byori. The Japanese Journal of Clinical Pathology. 2004;**52**(3):223-230

[20] Sun T, Cornejo K, Al-Turkmani M, Rao LV. Total prostate-specific antigen (tPSA) outperforms free PSA percentage (fPSA%) in detecting high-grade prostate carcinoma (PCa) in patients older than 60 years of age. North American Journal of Medicine and Science. 2019;**12**(1):7-13

[21] Lilja H. Biology of prostate-specific antigen. Urology. 2003;**62**(5 Suppl 1):27-33

[22] Christensson A, Björk T, Nilsson O, Dahlén U, Matikainen MT, Cockett AT, et al. Serum prostate specific antigen complexed to alpha 1-antichymotrypsin as an indicator of prostate cancer. The Journal of Urology. 1993;**150**(1):100-105

[23] Faria EF, Carvalhal GF, dos Reis RB, Tobias-Machado M, Vieira RA, Reis LO, et al. Use of low free to total PSA ratio in prostate cancer screening: Detection rates, clinical and pathological findings in Brazilian men with serum PSA levels <4.0 ng/mL. British Journal of Urology International. 2012;**110**(11 Pt B):E653-E657

[24] Omar J, Jaafar Z, Abdullah MR. A pilot study on percent free prostate specific antigen as an additional tool in prostate cancer screening. The Malaysian Journal of Medical Sciences. 2009;**16**(1):44-47

[25] Chen R, Xie L, Cai X, Huang Y, Zhou L, Ma L, et al. Percent free prostate-specific antigen for prostate cancer diagnosis in Chinese men with a PSA of 4.0-10.0 ng/mL: Results from the Chinese Prostate Cancer Consortium. Asian Journal of Urology. 2015;**2**(2):107-113

[26] Day JR, Jost M, Reynolds MA, Groskopf J, Rittenhouse H. PCA3: From basic molecular science to the clinical lab. Cancer Letters. 2011;**301**(1):1-6

[27] Auprich M, Augustin H, Budäus L, Kluth L, Mannweiler S, Shariat SF, et al. A comparative performance analysis of total prostate-specific antigen, percentage free prostate-specific antigen, prostate-specific antigen velocity and urinary prostate cancer gene 3 in the first, second and third repeat prostate biopsy. British Journal of Urology. 2012;**109**(11):1627-1635

[28] Merola R, Tomao L, Antenucci A, Sperduti I, Sentinelli S, Masi S, et al. PCA3 in prostate cancer and tumor aggressiveness detection on 407 high-risk patients: A National Cancer Institute experience. Journal of Experimental and Clinical Cancer Research. 2015;**34**(1):15. DOI: 10.1186/s13046-015-0127-8

[29] Simanek V, Topolcan O, Karlikova M, Dolejsova O, Fuchsova R, Kinkorova J, et al. Stability of total prostate-specific antigen and free prostate-specific antigen after 10 years' storage. The International Journal of Biological Markers. 2018; **33**(4):463-466

[30] Leyten GH, Hessels D, Jannink SA, Smit FP, de Jong H, Cornel EB, et al. Prospective multicentre evaluation of PCA3 and TMPRSS2-ERG gene fusions as diagnostic and prognostic urinary biomarkers for prostate cancer. European Urology. 2014;**65**:534-542

[31] Konety B, Zappala SM, Parekh DJ, Osterhout D, Schock J, Chudler RM, et al. The 4Kscore® test reduces prostate biopsy rates in community and academic urology practices. Reviews in Urology. 2015;**17**(4):231-240

[32] Matuszczak M, Schalken JA, Salagierski M. Prostate cancer liquid biopsy biomarkers' clinical utility in diagnosis and prognosis. Cancers. 2021;**13**(13):3373. DOI: 10.3390/cancers13133373

[33] Spratt DE, Yousefi K, Deheshi S, Ross AE, Den RB, Schaeffer EM, et al. Individual patient-level meta-Analysis of the performance of the decipher genomic classifier in high-risk men after prostatectomy to predict development of metastatic disease. Journal of Clinical Oncology. 2017;**35**(18):1991-1998

[34] Dalela D, Santiago-Jiménez M, Yousefi K, Karnes RJ, Ross AE, Den RB, et al. Genomic classifier augments the role of pathological features in identifying optimal candidates for adjuvant radiation therapy in patients with prostate cancer: Development and internal validation of a multivariable prognostic model. Journal of Clinical Oncology. 2017;**35**(18):1982-1990

[35] Gore JL, du Plessis M, Santiago-Jiménez M, Yousefi K, Thompson DJS, Karsh L, et al. Decipher test impacts decision making among patients considering adjuvant and salvage treatment after radical prostatectomy: Interim results from the Multicenter Prospective PRO-IMPACT study. Cancer. 2017;**123**(15):2850-2859

[36] Den RB, Feng FY, Showalter TN, Mishra MV, Trabulsi EJ, Lallas CD, et al. Genomic prostate cancer classifier predicts biochemical failure and metastases in patients after postoperative radiation therapy. International Journal of Radiation Oncology, Biology, Physics. 2014;**89**(5):1038-1046

[37] Van den Broeck T, Moris L, Gevaert T, Tosco L, Smeets E, Fishbane N, et al. Validation of the Decipher Test for predicting distant metastatic recurrence in men with high-risk non-metastatic prostate cancer 10 years after surgery. European Urology Oncology. 2019;**2**(5):589-596

[38] Kim HL, Li P, Huang HC, Deheshi S, Marti T, Knudsen B, et al. Validation of the Decipher Test for predicting adverse pathology in candidates for prostate cancer active surveillance. Prostate Cancer Prostatic Diseases. 2019;**22**(3):399-405

[39] Vince RA Jr, Jiang R, Qi J, Tosoian JJ, Takele R, Feng FY, et al. Impact of Decipher Biopsy testing on clinical outcomes in localized prostate cancer in a prospective statewide collaborative. Prostate Cancer Prostatic Disease. 2021. DOI: 10.1038/s41391-021-00428-y [online publication]

[40] White C, Staff I, McLaughlin T, Tortora J, Pinto K, Gangakhedkar A, et al. Does post prostatectomy decipher score predict biochemical recurrence and

impact care? World Journal of Urology. 2021;**39**(9):3281-3286

[41] Jairath NK, Dal Pra A, Vince R Jr, Dess RT, Jackson WC, Tosoian JJ, et al. A systematic review of the evidence for the decipher genomic classifier in prostate cancer. European Urology. 2021;**79**(3):374-383

[42] Marascio J, Spratt DE, Zhang J, Trabulsi EJ, Le T, Sedzorme WS, et al. Prospective study to define the clinical utility and benefit of Decipher testing in men following prostatectomy. Prostate Cancer and Prostatic Diseases. 2019;**23**(2):295-302

[43] Cullen J, Rosner IL, Brand TC, Zhang N, Tsiatis AC, Moncur J, et al. A biopsy-based 17-gene genomic prostate score predicts recurrence after radical prostatectomy and adverse surgical pathology in a racially diverse population of men with clinically low- and intermediate-risk prostate cancer. European Urology. 2015;**68**:123-131

[44] Cullen J, Lynch JA, Klein EA, Van Den Eeden SK, Carroll PR, Mohler JL, et al. Multicenter comparison of 17-Gene genomic prostate score as a predictor of outcomes in African American and Caucasian American men with clinically localized prostate cancer. Journal of Urology. 2021;**205**(4):1047-1054

[45] Murphy AB, Carbunaru S, Nettey OS, Gornbein C, Dixon MA, Macias V, et al. A 17-Gene panel genomic prostate score has similar predictive accuracy for adverse pathology at radical prostatectomy in African American and European American men. Urology. 2020;**142**:166-173

[46] Kornberg Z, Cooperberg MR, Cowan JE, Chan JM, Shinohara K, Simko JP, et al. A 17-Gene Genomic Prostate Score as a predictor of adverse pathology in men on active surveillance. Journal of Urology. 2019;**202**(4):702-709

[47] Lynch JA, Rothney MP, Salup RR, Ercole CE, Mathur SC, Duchene DA, et al. Improving risk stratification among veterans diagnosed with prostate cancer: Impact of the 17-gene prostate score assay. The American Journal of Managed Care. 2018;**24**(1 Suppl):S4-S10

[48] Chang EM, Punglia RS, Steinberg ML, Raldow AC. Cost effectiveness of the Oncotype DX Genomic Prostate Score for guiding treatment decisions in patients with early stage prostate cancer. Urology. 2019;**126**:89-95

[49] Partin AW, Van Neste L, Klein EA, Marks LS, Gee JR, Troyer DA, et al. Clinical validation of an epigenetic assay to predict negative histopathological results in repeat prostate biopsies. The Journal of Urology. 2014;**192**(4):1081-1087

[50] Waterhouse RL Jr, Van Neste L, Moses KA, Barnswell C, Silberstein JL, Jalkut M, et al. Evaluation of an epigenetic assay for predicting repeat prostate biopsy outcome in African American men. Urology. 2019;**128**:62-65

[51] Wojno KJ, Costa FJ, Cornell RJ, Small JD, Pasin E, Van Criekinge W, et al. Reduced rate of repeated prostate biopsies observed in ConfirmMDx clinical utility field study. American Health & Drug Benefits. 2014;**7**(3):129-134

[52] Blume-Jensen P, Berman DM, Rimm DL, Shipitsin M, Putzi M, Nifong TP, et al. Development and clinical validation of an in situ biopsy-based multimarker assay for risk stratification in prostate cancer. Clinical Cancer Research. 2015;**21**(11):2591-2600

[53] Garzon R, Calin GA, Croce CM. MicroRNAs in Cancer. Annual Review of Medicine. 2009;**60**:167-179

[54] Catalona WJ, Smith DS. Cancer recurrence and survival rates after anatomic radical retropubic prostatectomy for prostate cancer: Intermediate-term results. The Journal of Urology. 1998;**160**(6 Pt 2):2428-2434

[55] Khan MA, Sokoll LJ, Chan DW, Mangold LA, Mohr P, Mikolajczyk SD, et al. Clinical utility of proPSA and "Benign"s PSA when percent free PSA is less than 15%. Urology. 2004;**64**(6):1160-1164

[56] Yang J, Tang A, Zhang S, Sun X, Ming L. The age-specific reference intervals for tPSA, fPSA, and %fPSA in healthy Han ethnic male. Journal of Clinical Laboratory Analysis. 2017;**31**(4):e22062. DOI: 10.1002/jcla.22062

[57] Kim JH, Hong SK. Clinical utility of current biomarkers for prostate cancer detection. Investigative and Clinical Urology. 2021;**62**(1):1-13

[58] Fujita K, Nonomura N. Urinary biomarkers of prostate cancer. International Journal of Urology. 2018;**25**(9):770-779

[59] Schalken J, Interview with Jack Schalken. PCA3 and its use as a diagnostic test in prostate cancer. Interview by Christine McKillop. European Urology. 2006;**50**(1):153-154

[60] Hessels D, Schalken JA. The use of PCA3 in the diagnosis of prostate cancer. Nature Reviews Urology. 2009;**6**(5):255-261

[61] Bourdoumis A, Papatsoris AG, Chrisofos M, Efstathiou E, Skolarikos A, Deliveliotis C. The novel prostate cancer antigen 3 (PCA3) biomarker. International Brazilian Journal of Urology. 2010;**36**(6):665-669

[62] Salagierski M, Schalken JA. PCA3 and TMPRSS2-ERG: Promising biomarkers in prostate cancer diagnosis. Cancers (Basel). 2010;**2**(3):1432-1440

[63] Cui Y, Cao W, Li Q, Shen H, Liu C, Deng J, et al. Evaluation of prostate cancer antigen 3 for detecting prostate cancer: A systematic review and meta-analysis. Scientific Reports. 2016;**10**(6):25776. DOI: 10.1038/srep25776

[64] van Gils MP, Cornel EB, Hessels D, Peelen WP, Witjes JA, Mulders PF, et al. Molecular PCA3 diagnostics on prostatic fluid. The Prostate. 2007;**67**(8):881-887

[65] Wang T, Qu X, Jiang J, Gao P, Zhao D, Lian X, et al. Diagnostic significance of urinary long non-coding PCA3 RNA in prostate cancer. Oncotarget. 2017;**8**(35):58577-58586

[66] Gittelman MC, Hertzman B, Bailen J, Williams T, Koziol I, Henderson RJ, et al. PCA3 molecular urine test as a predictor of repeat prostate biopsy outcome in men with previous negative biopsies: A prospective multicenter clinical study. The Journal of Urology. 2013;**190**(1):64-69

[67] Ploussard G, Durand X, Xylinas E, Moutereau S, Radulescu C, Forgue A, et al. Prostate cancer antigen 3 score accurately predicts tumour volume and might help in selecting prostate cancer patients for active surveillance. European Urology. 2011;**59**(3):422-429

[68] Mistry K, Cable G. Meta-analysis of prostate-specific antigen and digital rectal examination as screening tests for prostate carcinoma. The Journal of the American Board of Family Practice. 2003;**16**(2):95-101

[69] Postma R, Schröder FH. Screening for prostate cancer. European Journal of Cancer. 2005;**41**(6):825-833

[70] Loeb S, Catalona WJ. The Prostate Health Index: A new test for the detection of prostate cancer. Therapeutic Advances in Urology. 2014;**6**(2):74-77

[71] Beckman CI. FDA Approves new blood test to improve prostate cancer detection [Internet]. 2012. https://www.prnewswire.com/news-releases/fda-approves-new-blood-test-to-improve-prostate-cancer-detection-160267195.html [Accessed 19 January 2022]

[72] Pecoraro V, Roli L, Plebani M, et al. Clinical utility of the (−2)proPSA and evaluation of the evidence: A systematic review. Clinical Chemistry and Laboratory Medicine. 2016;**54**(7):1123-1132

[73] Catalona WJ, Partin AW, Sanda MG, et al. A multicenter study of [−2] pro-prostate-specific antigen combined with prostate-specific antigen and free prostate-specific antigen for prostate cancer detection in the 2.0 to 10.0 ng/mL prostate-specific antigen range. Journal of Urology. 2011;**185**:1650-1655

[74] Loeb S, Sokoll L, Broyles D, Bangma C, van Schaik R, Klee G. Prospective multicenter evaluation of the Beckman Coulter Prostate Health Index using WHO calibration. Journal of Urology. 2013;**189**:1702-1706

[75] Zhang G, Li Y, Li C, Li N, Li Z, Zhou Q. Assessment on clinical value of prostate health index in the diagnosis of prostate cancer. Cancer Medicine. 2019;**8**:5089-5096

[76] Chang KN, Hu F, Zheng W, Kwan WW, Iam-Ting IP, Shrestha S, et al. Prostate health index for the diagnosis of prostate cancer in Asians in Macau with a PSA level of 4-10 μg/L. Zhonghua Nan Ke Xue. 2021;**27**(9):803-808

[77] Kim JY, Yu JH, Sung LH, Cho DY, Kim HJ, Yoo SJ. Usefulness of the prostate health index in predicting the presence and aggressiveness of prostate cancer among Korean men: A prospective observational study. BioMed Central Urology. 2021;**21**(1):131. DOI: 10.1186/s12894-021-00897-2

[78] Akdogan N, Aridogan IA, Izol V, Deger M, Gokalp F, Bayazit Y, et al. Use of the prostate health index in the detection of prostate cancer at all PSA levels (use of prostate health index in prostate cancer). International Journal of Clinical Practice. 2021;**75**(4):e13922. DOI: 10.1111/ijcp.13922

[79] Nandakumar V, Bornhorst JA, Algeciras-Schimnich A. Evaluation of Phi clinical performance for the detection of prostate cancer in routine clinical practice. Annals of Clinical and Laboratory Science. 2021;**51**(1):3-11

[80] Nahar B, Punnen S, Sjoberg D, Zappala SM, Parekh D. The 4Kscore to predict the grade and stage of prostate cancer in the radical prostatectomy specimen: Results from a multi-institutional prospective trial. Journal of Clinical Oncology. 2016;**34**(2 suppl):69-69. DOI: 10.1200/jco.2016.34.2

[81] Kim EH, Andriole GL, Crawford ED, Sjoberg DD, Assel M, Vickers AJ, et al. Detection of high grade prostate cancer among PLCO participants using a pre-specified 4-Kallikrein marker panel. The Journal of urology. 2017;**197**(4):1041-1047

[82] Hessels D, Smit FP, Verhaegh GW, Witjes JA, Cornel EB, Schalken JA. Detection of TMPRSS2-ERG fusion transcripts and prostate cancer antigen 3 in urinary sediments may improve diagnosis of prostate cancer. Clinical Cancer Research. 2007;**13**:5103-5108

[83] Eskra JN, Rabizadeh D, Pavlovich CP, Catalona WJ, Luo J. Approaches to

urinary detection of prostate cancer. Prostate Cancer and Prostatic Diseases. 2019;**22**:362-381

[84] St John J, Powell K, Conley-Lacomb MK, Chinni SR. TMPRSS2-ERG fusion gene expression in prostate tumor cells and its clinical and biological significance in prostate cancer progression. Journal of Cancer Science and Therapy. 2012;**4**:94-101

[85] Tomlins SA, Day JR, Lonigro RJ, Hovelson DH, Siddiqui J, Kunju LP, et al. Urine TMPRSS2:ERG Plus PCA3 for individualized prostate cancer risk assessment. European Urology. 2016;**70**:45-53

[86] Hermans KG, van Marion R, van Dekken H, Jenster G, van Weerden WM, Trapman J. TMPRSS2:ERG fusion by translocation or interstitial deletion is highly relevant in androgen-dependent prostate cancer, but is bypassed in late-stage androgen receptor-negative prostate cancer. Cancer Research. 2006;**66**:10658-10663

[87] Hossain D, Bostwick DG. Significance of the TMPRSS2:ERG gene fusion in prostate cancer. BJU international. 2013;**111**:834-835

[88] Salagierski M, Schalken JA. Molecular diagnosis of prostate cancer: PCA3 and TMPRSS2:ERG gene fusion. The Journal of Urology. 2012;**187**:795-801

[89] Song C, Chen H. Predictive significance of TMRPSS2-ERG fusion in prostate cancer: A meta-analysis. Cancer Cell International. 2018;**18**:177. DOI: 10.1186/s12935-018-0672-2

[90] Clark J, Cooper C. ETS gene fusions in prostate cancer. Nature Reviews Urology. 2009;**6**:429-439

[91] Kohaar I, Petrovics G, Srivastava S. A rich array of prostate cancer molecular biomarkers: Opportunities and challenges. International Journal of Molecular Sciences. 2019;**20**:1813. DOI: org/10.3390/ijms20081813

[92] Rice KR, Chen Y, Ali A, Whitman EJ, Blase A, Ibrahim M, et al. Evaluation of the ETS-related gene mRNA in urine for the detection of prostate cancer. Clinical Cancer Research. 2010;**16**:1572-1576

[93] Salami SS, Schmidt F, Laxman B, Regan MM, Rickman DS, Scherr D, et al. Combining urinary detection of TMPRSS2:ERG and PCA3 with serum PSA to predict diagnosis of prostate cancer. Urologic Oncology. 2013;**31**:566-571

[94] Tomlins SA, Aubin SM, Siddiqui J, Lonigro RJ, Sefton-Miller L, Miick S, et al. Urine TMPRSS2:ERG fusion transcript stratifies prostate cancer risk in men with elevated serum PSA. Science Translational Medicine. 2011;**3**(94):94ra72. DOI: org/10.1126/scitranslmed.3001970

[95] Leyten GH, Hessels D, Smit FP, Jannink SA, de Jong H, Melchers WJ, et al. Identification of a candidate gene panel for the early diagnosis of prostate cancer. Clinical Cancer Research. 2015;**21**:3061-3070

[96] Eyrich NW, Morgan TM, Tosoian JJ. Biomarkers for detection of clinically significant prostate cancer: Contemporary clinical data and future directions. Translational Andrology and Urology. 2021;**10**:3091-3103

[97] McCabe CD, Spyropoulos DD, Martin D, Moreno CS. Genome-wide analysis of the homeobox C6 transcriptional network in prostate cancer. Cancer Research. 2008;**68**(6):1988-1996

[98] Ramachandran S, Liu P, Young A, Yin-Goen O, Lim SD, Laycock N, et al.

Loss of HOXC6 expression induces apoptosis in prostate cancer cells. Oncogene. 2005;**24**:188-198

[99] Liang M, Sun Y, Yang HL, Zhang B, Wen J, Shi BK. DLX1, a binding protein of beta-catenin, promoted the growth and migration of prostate cancer cells. Experimental Cell Res. 2018;**363**:26-32

[100] Van Neste L, Hendriks RJ, Dijkstra S, Trooskens G, Cornel EB, Jannink SA, et al. Detection of high-grade prostate cancer using a urinary molecular biomarker-based risk score. European Urology. 2016;**70**:740-748

[101] Govers TM, Hessels D, Vlaeminck-Guillem V, Schmitz-Dräger BJ, Stief CG, Martinez-Ballesteros C, et al. Cost-effectiveness of SelectMDx for prostate cancer in four European countries: A comparative modeling study. Prostate Cancer and Prostatic Diseases. 2019;**22**:101-109

[102] Haese A, Trooskens G, Steyaert S, Hessels D, Brawer M, Vlaeminck-Guillem V, et al. Multicenter optimization and validation of a 2-Gene mRNA urine test for detection of clinically significant prostate cancer before initial prostate biopsy. The Journal of Urology. 2019;**202**(2):256-263

[103] Klein EA, Cooperberg MR, Magi-Galluzzi C, Simko JP, Falzarano SM, Maddala T, et al. A 17-gene assay to predict prostate cancer aggressiveness in the context of Gleason grade heterogeneity, tumor multi-focality, and biopsy under-sampling. European Urology. 2014;**66**:550-560

[104] Van Den Eeden SK, Lu R, Zhang N, Quesenberry CP Jr, Shan J, Han JS, et al. A biopsy-based 17-gene genomic prostate score as a predictor of metastases and prostate cancer death in surgically treated men with clinically

localized disease. European Urology. 2018;**73**:129-138

[105] Brooks MA, Thomas L, Magi-Galluzzi C, Li J, Crager MR, Lu R, et al. GPS Assay association with long-term cancer outcomes: Twenty-year risk of distant metastasis and prostate cancer-specific mortality. JCO Precision. Oncology. 2021;**5**. DOI: 10.1200/PO.20.00325

[106] Lin DW, Zheng Y, McKenney JK, Brown MD, Lu R, Crager M, et al. 17-Gene Genomic Prostate Score Test results in the Canary Prostate Active Surveillance Study (PASS) Cohort. Journal of Clinical Oncology. 2020;**38**(14):1549-1557

[107] Marascio J, Spratt DE, Zhang J, Trabulsi EJ, Le T, Sedzorme WS, et al. Prospective study to define the clinical utility and benefit of Decipher testing in men following prostatectomy. Prostate Cancer Prostatic Disease. 2020;**23**(2):295-302

[108] Srivastava A, Suy S, Collins SP, Kumar D. Circulating microRNA as biomarkers: An update in prostate cancer. Molecular and Cellular Pharmacology. 2011;**3**(3):115-124

[109] Lobo JM, Trifiletti DM, Sturz VN, Dicker AP, Buerki C, Davicioni E, et al. Cost-effectiveness of the Decipher Genomic Classifier to guide individualized decisions for early radiation therapy after prostatectomy for prostate cancer. Clinical Genitourinary Cancer. 2017;**15**(3):e299-e309

[110] Blute ML, Damaschke NA, Jarrard DF. The epigenetics of prostate cancer diagnosis and prognosis. Current Opinion in Urology. 2015;**25**(1):83-88

[111] Stewart GD, Van Neste L, Delvenne P, Delrée P, Delga A, McNeill SA, et al. Clinical utility of

an epigenetic assay to detect occult prostate cancer in histopathologically negative biopsies: Results of the MATLOC Study. The Journal of Urology. 2013;**189**(3):1110-1116

[112] Shipitsin M, Small C, Choudhury S, Giladi E, Friedlander S, Nardone J, et al. Identification of proteomic biomarkers predicting prostate cancer aggressiveness and lethality despite biopsy-sampling error. British Journal of Cancer. 2014;**111**(6):1201-1212

[113] Shipitsin M, Small C, Giladi E, Siddiqui S, Choudhury S, Hussain S, et al. Automated quantitative multiplex immunofluorescence in situ imaging identifies phospho-S6 and phospho-PRAS40 as predictive protein biomarkers for prostate cancer lethality. Proteome Science. 2014;**12**:40 DOI: 10.1186/1477-5956-12-40

[114] Luu HN, Lin HY, Sørensen KD, Ogunwobi OO, Kumar N, Chornokur G, et al. miRNAs associated with prostate cancer risk and progression. BMC Urology. 2017;**17**(1):18. DOI: 10.1186/s12894-017-0206-6

[115] Jin W, Fei X, Wang X, Chen F, S ong Y. Circulating miRNAs as biomarkers for prostate cancer diagnosis in subjects with benign prostatic hyperplasia. Journal of Immunology Research. 2020;**2020**:5873056. DOI: 10.1155/2020/5873056

[116] Ibrahim NH, Abdellateif MS, Kassem SH, Abd El Salam MA, El Gammal MM. Diagnostic significance of miR-21, miR-141, miR-18a and miR-221 as novel biomarkers in prostate cancer among Egyptian patients. Andrologia. 2019;**51**(10):e13384. DOI: org/10.1111/and.13384

[117] Cai B, Peng JH. Increased expression of miR-494 in serum of patients with prostate cancer and its potential diagnostic value. Clinical Laboratory. 2019;**65**(8):10.7754. DOI: 10.7754/Clin.Lab.2019.190422

[118] Kolluru V, Chandrasekaran B, Tyagi A, Dervishi A, Ankem M, Yan X, et al. miR-301a expression: Diagnostic and prognostic marker for prostate cancer. Urologic Oncology. 2018;**36**(11):503.e9-503.e15. DOI: org/10.1016/j.urolonc.2018.07.014

[119] Wang J, Ye H, Zhang D, Hu Y, Yu X, Wang L, et al. MicroRNA-410-5p as a potential serum biomarker for the diagnosis of prostate cancer. Cancer Cell International. 2016;**16**:12. DOI: 10.1186/s12935-016-0285-6

[120] Lieb V, Weigelt K, Scheinost L, Fischer K, Greither T, Marcou M, et al. Serum levels of miR-320 family members are associated with clinical parameters and diagnosis in prostate cancer patients. Oncotarget. 2017;**9**(12):10402-10416

[121] Sun X, Yang Z, Zhang Y, He J, Wang F, Su P, et al. Prognostic implications of tissue and serum levels of microRNA-128 in human prostate cancer. International Journal of Clinical and Experimental Pathology. 2015;**8**(7):8394-8401

[122] Srivastava A, Goldberger H, Dimtchev A, Marian C, Soldin O, Li X, et al. Circulatory miR-628-5p is down-regulated in prostate cancer patients. Tumour Biology. 2014;**35**(5):4867-4873

[123] Lyu J, Zhao L, Wang F, Ji J, Cao Z, Xu H, et al. Discovery and validation of serum microRNAs as early diagnostic biomarkers for prostate cancer in Chinese population. BioMed Research International. 2019;**2019**:9306803. DOI: 10.1155/2019/9306803

[124] Al-Kafaji G, Said HM, Alam MA, Al Naieb ZT. Blood-based microRNAs as diagnostic biomarkers to discriminate

localized prostate cancer from benign prostatic hyperplasia and allow cancer-risk stratification. Oncology Letters. 2018;**16**(1):1357-1365

[125] Zedan AH, Hansen TF, Assenholt J, Pleckaitis M, Madsen JS, Osther PJS. microRNA expression in tumour tissue and plasma in patients with newly diagnosed metastatic prostate cancer. Tumour Biology 2018;**40**(5):1010428. DOI: 10.1177/1010428318775864

[126] Martínez-González LJ, Sánchez-Conde V, González-Cabezuelo JM, Antunez-Rodríguez A, Andrés-León E, Robles-Fernandez I, et al. Identification of microRNAs as viable aggressiveness biomarkers for prostate cancer. Biomedicine. 2021;**9**(6):646. DOI: org/10.3390/biomedicines9060646

[127] Zedan AH, Osther P, Assenholt J, Madsen JS, Hansen TF. Circulating miR-141 and miR-375 are associated with treatment outcome in metastatic castration resistant prostate cancer. Scientific Reports. 2020;**10**(1):227. DOI: org/10.1038/s41598-019-57101-7

[128] Guo X, Han T, Hu P, Guo X, Zhu C, Wang Y, et al. Five microRNAs in serum as potential biomarkers for prostate cancer risk assessment and therapeutic intervention. International Urology and Nephrology. 2018;**50**(12):2193-2200

[129] Liu R, Olkhov-Mitsel E, Jeyapala R, Zhao F, Commisso K, Klotz L, et al. Assessment of serum microRNA biomarkers to predict reclassification of prostate cancer in patients on active surveillance. The Journal of Urology. 2018;**199**(6):1475-1481

[130] Souza MF, Kuasne H, Barros-Filho MC, Cilião HL, Marchi FA, Fuganti PE, et al. Circulating mRNAs and miRNAs as candidate markers for the diagnosis and prognosis of prostate

cancer. PLoS One. 2017;**12**(9):e0184094. DOI: org/10.1371/journal.pone.0184094

[131] Abramovic I, Vrhovec B, Skara L, Vrtaric A, Nikolac Gabaj N, Kulis T, et al. MiR-182-5p and miR-375-3p have higher performance than PSA in discriminating prostate cancer from benign prostate hyperplasia. Cancers (Basel). 2021;**13**(9):2068. DOI: 10.3390/cancers13092068

[132] Bidarra D, Constâncio V, Barros-Silva D, Ramalho-Carvalho J, Moreira-Barbosa C, Antunes L, et al. Circulating MicroRNAs as biomarkers for prostate cancer detection and metastasis development prediction. Frontiers in Oncology. 2019;**9**:900. DOI: org/10.3389/fonc.2019.00900

[133] Duca RB, Massillo C, Dalton GN, Farré PL, Graña KD, Gardner K, et al. MiR-19b-3p and miR-101-3p as potential biomarkers for prostate cancer diagnosis and prognosis. American Journal of Cancer Research. 2021;**11**(6):2802-2820

[134] Rajendiran S, Maji S, Haddad A, Lotan Y, Nandy RR, Vishwanatha JK, et al. MicroRNA-940 as a potential serum biomarker for prostate cancer. Frontiers. Oncology. 2021;**11**:628094. DOI: 10.3389/fonc.2021.628094

[135] Huang Z, Zhang L, Yi X, Yu X. Diagnostic and prognostic values of tissue hsa-miR-30c and hsa-miR-203 in prostate carcinoma. Tumour Bioliogy. 2016;**37**(4):4359-4365

[136] Paziewska A, Mikula M, Dabrowska M, Kulecka M, Goryca K, Antoniewicz A, et al. Candidate diagnostic miRNAs that can detect cancer in prostate biopsy. The Prostate. 2018;**78**(3):178-185

[137] Li T, Sun X, Liu Y. miR-27b expression in diagnosis and evaluation prognosis of prostate

cancer. International Journal of Clinical and Experimental Pathology. 2017;**10**(12):11415-11424

[138] Zhu C, Hou X, Zhu J, Jiang C, Wei W. Expression of miR-30c and miR-29b in prostate cancer and its diagnostic significance. Oncology Letters. 2018;**16**(3):3140-3144

[139] Richardsen E, Andersen S, Al-Saad S, Rakaee M, Nordby Y, Pedersen MI, et al. Low expression of miR-424-3p is highly correlated with clinical failure in prostate cancer. Scientific Reports. 2019;**9**(1):10662. DOI: org/10.1038/s41598-019-47234-0

[140] Zhang J, Li S, Li L, Li M, Guo C, Yao J, et al. Exosome and exosomal microRNA: Trafficking, sorting, and function. Genomics Proteomics & Bioinformatics. 2015;**13**(1):17-24

[141] Stoen MJ, Andersen S, Rakaee M, Pedersen MI, Ingebriktsen LM, Donnem T, et al. Overexpression of miR-20a-5p in tumor epithelium is an independent negative prognostic indicator in prostate cancer - A multi-Institutional study. Cancers. 2021;**13**(16):4096. DOI: org/10.3390/cancers13164096

[142] García-Magallanes N, Beltran-Ontiveros SA, Leal-León EA, Luque-Ortega F, Romero-Quintana JG, Osuna-Ramirez I, et al. Under-expression of circulating miR-145-5p and miR-133a-3p are associated with breast cancer and immuno-histochemical markers. Journal of Cancer Research and Therapeutics. 2020;**16**(6):1223-1228

[143] Wang Y, Zhang Q, Guo B, Feng J, Zhao D. miR-1231 is downregulated in prostate cancer with prognostic and functional implications. Oncology Research and Treatment. 2020;**43**(3):78-86

[144] Laursen EB, Fredsøe J, Schmidt L, Strand SH, Kristensen H, Rasmussen A, et al. Elevated miR-615-3p expression predicts adverse clinical outcome and promotes proliferation and migration of prostate cancer cells. The American Journal of Pathology. 2019;**189**(12):2377-2388

[145] Bi CW, Zhang GY, Bai Y, Zhao B, Yang H. Increased expression of miR-153 predicts poor prognosis for patients with prostate cancer. Medicine. 2019;**98**(36):e16705. DOI: org/10.1097/MD.0000000000016705

[146] Hashimoto Y, Shiina M, Dasgupta P, Kulkarni P, Kato T, Wong RK, et al. Upregulation of miR-130b contributes to risk of poor prognosis and racial disparity in African-American prostate cancer. Cancer Prevention Research. 2019;**12**(9):585-598

[147] Das DK, Ogunwobi OO. A novel microRNA-1207-3p/FNDC1/FN1/AR regulatory pathway in prostate cancer. RNA & Disease (Houston, Tex.). 2017;**4**(1):e1503

[148] Damodaran C, Das TP, Papu John AM, Suman S, Kolluru V, Morris TJ, et al. miR-301a expression: A prognostic marker for prostate cancer. Urologic Oncology. 2016;**34**(8):336.e13-336.e20. DOI: org/10.1016/j.urolonc.2016.03.009

[149] Doldi V, El Bezawy R, Zaffaroni N. MicroRNAs as epigenetic determinants of treatment response and potential therapeutic targets in prostate cancer. Cancers. 2021;**13**(10):2380. DOI: org/10.3390/cancers13102380

[150] Skotland T, Hessvik NP, Sandvig K, Llorente A. Exosomal lipid composition and the role of ether lipids and phosphoinositides in exosome biology. Journal Lipid Research. 2019;**60**:9-18

[151] Cappello F, Logozzi M, Campanella C, Bavisotto CC, Marcilla A, Properzi F, et al. Exosome levels in human body fluids: A tumor marker by themselves? European Journal of Pharmaceutical Sciences. 2017;**96**:93-98

[152] Gulei D, Petrut B, Tigu AB, Onaciu A, Fischer-Fodor E, Atanasov AG, et al. Exosomes at a glance - common nominators for cancer hallmarks and novel diagnosis tools. Critical Reviews in Biochemistry and Molecular Biology. 2018;**53**(5):564-577

[153] Gao Z, Pang B, Li J, Gao N, Fan T, Li Y. Emerging role of exosomes in liquid biopsy for monitoring prostate cancer invasion and metastasis. Frontiers in Cell Development Biology. 2021;**9**:679527. DOI: 10.3389/fcell.2021.679527

[154] Lorenc T, Klimczyk K, Michalczewska I, Słomka M, Kubiak-Tomaszewska G, Olejarz W. Exosomes in prostate cancer diagnosis, prognosis and therapy. International Journal of Molecular Sciences. 2020;**21**(6):2118. DOI: 10.3390/ijms21062118

[155] Li C, Ni YQ, Xu H, Xiang QY, Zhao Y, Zhan JK, et al. Roles and mechanisms of exosomal non-coding RNAs in human health and diseases. Signal Transduction and Targeted Therapy. 2021;**6**(1):383. DOI: 10.1038/s41392-021-00779-x

[156] Luo R, Liu M, Yang Q, Cheng H, Yang H, Li M, et al. Emerging diagnostic potential of tumor-derived exosomes. Journal of Cancer. 2021;**12**(16):5035-5045

[157] Li W, Dong Y, Wang KJ, Deng Z, Zhang W, Shen HF. Plasma exosomal miR-125a-5p and miR-141-5p as non-invasive biomarkers for prostate cancer. Neoplasma. 2020;**67**(6):1314-1318

[158] Huang X, Yuan T, Liang M, Du M, Xia S, Dittmar R, et al. Exosomal miR-1290 and miR-375 as prognostic markers in castration-resistant prostate cancer. European Urology. 2015;**67**(1):33-41

[159] Li Z, Ma YY, Wang J, Zeng XF, Li R, Kang W, et al. Exosomal microRNA-141 is upregulated in the serum of prostate cancer patients. OncoTargets and Therapy. 2015;**9**:139-148

[160] Bhagirath D, Yang TL, Bucay N, Sekhon K, Majid S, Shahryari V, et al. microRNA-1246 is an exosomal biomarker for aggressive prostate cancer. Cancer Research. 2018;**78**(7):1833-1844

[161] Xu Y, Lou J, Yu M, Jiang Y, Xu H, Huang Y, et al. Urinary exosomes diagnosis of urological tumors: A systematic review and meta-analysis. Frontiers in Oncology. 2021;**11**:734587. DOI: 10.3389/fonc.2021.734587

[162] Shin S, Park YH, Jung SH, Jang SH, Kim MY, Lee JY, et al. Urinary exosome microRNA signatures as a noninvasive prognostic biomarker for prostate cancer. NPJ Genomic Medicine. 2021;**6**(1):45. DOI: 10.1038/s41525-021-00212-w

[163] Wani S, Kaul D, Mavuduru RS, Kakkar N, Bhatia A. Urinary-exosomal miR-2909: A novel pathognomonic trait of prostate cancer severity. Journal of Biotechnology. 2017;**259**:135-139

[164] Lee J, Kwon MH, Kim JA, Rhee WJ. Detection of exosome miRNAs using molecular beacons for diagnosing prostate cancer. Artificial Cells, Nanomedicine and Biotechnology. 2018;**46**(3):S52-S63

[165] Kim MY, Shin H, Moon HW, Park YH, Park J, Lee JY. Urinary exosomal microRNA profiling in intermediate-risk prostate cancer. Scientific Reports. 2021;**11**(1):7355. DOI: 10.1038/s41598-021-86785-z

[166] McDunn JE, Li Z, Adam KP, Neri BP, Wolfert RL, Milburn MV, et al. Metabolomic signatures of aggressive prostate cancer. The Prostate. 2013;**73**:1547-1560

[167] Saylor PJ, Karoly ED, Smith MR. Prospective study of changes in the metabolomics profiles of men during their first three months of androgen deprivation therapy for prostate cancer. Clinical Cancer Research. 2012;**18**:3677-3685

[168] Sreekumar A, Poisson LM, Rajendiran TM, Khan AP, Cao Q, Yu J, et al. Metabolomic profiles delineate potential role for sarcosine in prostate cancer progression. Nature 2009;**457**(7231):910-914

[169] Sroka WD, Boughton BA, Reddy P, Roessner U, Słupski P, Jarzemski P, et al. Determination of amino acids in urine of patients with prostate cancer and benign prostate growth. European Journal of Cancer Prevention. 2017;**26**(2):131-134

[170] Parr RL, Mills J, Harbottle A, Creed JM, Crewdson G, Reguly B, et a l. Mitochondria, prostate cancer, and biopsy sampling error. Discovery Medicine. 2013;**15**(83):213-220

[171] Talukdar S, Emdad L, Das SK, Sarkar D, Fisher PB. Evolving strategies for therapeutically targeting cancer stem cells. Advances in Cancer Research. 2016;**131**:159-191

[172] Robinson K, Creed J, Reguly B, Powell C, Wittock R, Klein D, et al. Accurate prediction of repeat prostate biopsy outcomes by a mitochondrial DNA deletion assay. Prostate Cancer and Prostatic Diseases. 2010;**13**(2):126-131

[173] Legisi L, DeSa E, Qureshi MN. Use of the prostate core mitomic test in repeated biopsy decision-making: Real-world assessment of clinical utility in a multicenter patient population. American Health & Drug Benefits. 2016;**9**(9):497-502

[174] Hillyar C, Rizki H, Abbassi O, Miles-Dua S, Clayton G, Gandamihardja T, et al. Correlation between oncotype DX, PREDICT and the Nottingham Prognostic Index: Implications for the management of early breast cancer. Cureus. 2020;**12**(4):e7552. DOI: 10.7759/cureus.7552

[175] Moustafa AA, Kim H, Albeltagy RS, El-Habit OH, Abdel-Mageed AB. MicroRNAs in prostate cancer: From function to biomarker discovery. Experimental Biology and Medicine (Maywood, N.J.). 2018;**243**(10):817-825

[176] Ludwig N, Whiteside TL, Reichert TE. Challenges in exosome isolation and analysis in health and disease. International Journal of Molecular Science. 2019;**20**(19):4684. DOI: 10.3390/ijms20194684

[177] Hodges KB, Bachert E, Cheng L. Prostate cancer biomarkers: Current status. Critical Reviews in Oncogenesis. 2017;**22**(5-6):253-269. DOI: org/10.1615/CritRevOncog.2017020500

[178] Velonas VM, Woo HH, dos Remedios CG, Assinder SJ. Current status of biomarkers for prostate cancer. International Journal of Molecular Sciences. 2013;**14**(6):11034-11060

[179] Jamaspishvili T, Kral M, Khomeriki I, Student V, Kolar Z, Bouchal J. Urine markers in monitoring for prostate cancer. Prostate Cancer and Prostatic Diseases. 2010;**13**(1):12-19

[180] Wu D, Ni J, Beretov J, Cozzi P, Willcox M, Wasinger V, et al. Urinary biomarkers in prostate cancer detection and monitoring progression. Critical Reviews in Oncology/Hematology. 2017;**118**:15-26

[181] Malik A, Srinivasan S, Batra J. A new era of prostate cancer precision medicine. Frontiers in Oncology. 2019;**9**:1263. DOI: 10.3389/fonc.2019.01263

[182] Clinton TN, Bagrodia A, Lotan Y, Margulis V, Raj GV, Woldu SL. Tissue-based biomarkers in prostate cancer. Expert Rev Precis Med Drug Dev. 2017;**2**(5):249-260

[183] Hennigan ST, Trostel SY, Terrigino NT, Voznesensky OS, Schaefer RJ, Whitlock NC, et al. Low abundance of circulating tumor DNA in localized prostate cancer. JCO Precision Oncology. 2019;**3**. PO.19.00176. DOI: 10.1200/PO.19.00176

[184] Tukachinsky H, Madison RW, Chung JH, Gjoerup OV, Severson EA, Dennis L, et al. Genomic analysis of circulating tumor DNA in 3,334 patients with advanced prostate cancer identifies targetable BRCA alterations and AR resistance mechanisms. Clinical Cancer Research. 2021;**27**(11):3094-3105

[185] McKiernan J, Donovan MJ, O'Neill V, Bentink S, Noerholm M, Belzer S, et al. A novel urine exosome gene expression assay to predict high-grade prostate cancer at initial biopsy. JAMA Oncology. 2016;**2**:882-889

Section 2

The Importance of Cancer Registries

Chapter 6

The Role of Registration in Cancer Control and Prevention

Yelda A. Leal

Abstract

Cancer is one of the major causes of morbidity and mortality in the world, with 18.1 million new cases and 9.6 million deaths, and an estimated prevalence during the last 5 years of 43.8 million persons with the disease, according to 2018 World Health Organization (WHO) report. Disparities between developed and developing countries have been documented—nearly 57% of cancer cases (8 million) and 65% of cancer deaths (5.3 million) occurred in developing countries. Although more cases are detected in countries with a high or very high human development index, mortality rates are similar in both low-to-middle-income countries and high-to-very high-income countries. The global picture of the impact of cancer worldwide can only be calculated from registry data, which allow for estimations of the burden of cancer for different geographic areas, as well as for the fundamental role in cancer control and prevention.

Keywords: Cancer, registration, population, bioinformatics, prevention, control

1. Introduction

Noncommunicable diseases (NCDs), including cancer, are the leading causes of preventable and premature death, killing 40 million persons each year and accounting for about 70% of all deaths globally. Some 15 million of those deaths include people between 30 and 69 years of age, and more than 80% of these premature deaths occur in low-income and middle-income countries (LMIC); thus, NCDs are important and growing causes of health inequalities and inequities [1, 2].

Cancer remains a huge and leading cause of morbidity and mortality worldwide, with an annual incidence of 18.1 million new cases, and it is the second most common cause of death globally, accounting for an estimated 9.6 million deaths in 2018.

The burden of cancer is rising globally, but not equally; the greatest impact of cancer and the fastest increase in the cancer burden over the coming decades is projected to be in LMIC [3].

Controlling cancer is a multifaceted issue that requires multimodel solutions; one of the main solutions is the establishment of a cancer-control plan to overcome the growing cancer burden. The World Health Organization (WHO) defines the national cancer control plan (NCCP) as a public health program designed to reduce the incidence and mortality of the disease through the systematic and equitable implementation of evidence-based strategies for prevention, early detection, treatment, palliation, and to improve the quality of life of cancer patients, through the best use of available resources. Cancer registration is the priority issue for data-based evidence, which is essential for determining the cancer burden [2].

The burden of cancer is solely measured by cancer registration through the collecting of information on new cases (incidence). Cancer incidence by type has been included as a core indicator in the WHO-Global Monitoring Framework for the Prevention and Control of NCD, and the latter was reaffirmed at the recent 70th World Health Assembly [4, 5].

Cancer registration is much more than an epidemiological center; the surveillance of cancer incidence is quite different due to the complexity of cancer, which is not a single disease but rather a distinct entity that varies biologically, clinically, and epidemiologically. Many cancers are complex and heterogeneous in their characteristics, with hundreds of histological and biological subtypes. Given the diversity of cancer types in different geographic areas, it is necessary to base cancer-control activities on customized, individualized cancer profiles obtained through cancer registries, since each area has different circumstances and needs [6, 7].

Cancer registries provide the cancer-information patterns essential for planning and evaluating health services for the prevention and control of cancer. These registries comprise the main issue in terms of the effectiveness of health systems, public health interventions, and survivorship in order to assess treatment effectiveness, as well as for the primary prevention, early detection, screening, and treatment of cancer. Hence, cancer registration plays an essential role in the planning and evaluation of effective control and prevention policies [8].

2. Cancer registration

The cancer burden is rising globally, exerting a significant strain on populations and health systems at all income levels. The increasing number of cancer cases observed during the last decades is due in part to the epidemiological transition that took place worldwide, resulting mainly from the net growth of the population, the aging effect, and changing fertility rates, increased longevity, and changing lifestyles [9–11].

The differing cancer profiles in individual countries and between regions indicate marked geographic diversity, due to the distribution of patterns that implicate environmental determinants, lifestyles, occupation, physical activities, and other cancer risk factors. Variations in the prevalence of cancer risk factors influence the different cancer profiles between the different geographic areas because these factors are generally present in different magnitudes across different populations. For instance, infection-related and poverty-related cancers are common in developing countries, whereas in high-income countries, the cancer profile is most often associated with lifestyle. However, the cancer burden is greatest in low- and middle-income countries (LMIC), where approximately 75% of cancer deaths occur and where the number of cancer cases is rising most rapidly [10–13].

Global cancer control has been a growing priority for the authorities; for instance, WHO, in a joint effort with the World Health Assembly, the United Nations Agenda (UN), and local authorities, have made a commitment to global cancer control through the Global Cancer Plan on the Prevention and Control of NCD, in the 2030 United Nations Agenda for Sustainable Development Goals (SDG). One of the most important cutting-edge actions taken is that of the 2017-World Health Assembly

Resolution 70.12 on cancer prevention and control. This is an integrated approach that ensures access to treatment and care, palliative and survivorship care, and comprehensive data collection through robust cancer registries, because the incidence by cancer type is a core indicator of progress within the WHO-Global Monitoring Framework for NCD [1, 4, 12].

Accordingly, short- and long-term recommendations for tackling the rising cancer burden include the implementation of the national cancer control plan (NCCP). Thus, strategies for addressing the global cancer burden must be tailored to the local reality; the strategy must account for a country's most frequent cancer type and be tackled according to the country's available resources. Hence, to allocate resources properly, accurate and comprehensive cancer registries are essential for providing information on the cancer burden in the country. Therefore, all of the decisions involved must be based on the best available evidence and accurate epidemiological data addressed within the national cancer control plan [2, 12].

Cancer registries collect data on cancer cases over time. The main purpose of the cancer registry is to collect data continuously and systematically and to classify information on all cancer cases from various data sources in a defined area, in order to produce statistics for providing a framework for assessing and controlling the impact of cancer on the community, through estimating the current cancer burden, examining recent trends, and predicting their probable future evolution. The scale and profile of cancer can be evaluated in terms of incidence and mortality, but other dimensions are often considered, including prevalence, person-years-of-life-lost, and quality- or disability-adjusted life years. An appraisal of the current situation provides a framework for action, and cancer-control planning should include the establish-ment of explicit targets, which permits the success or otherwise of the interventions to be monitored [14, 15].

Cancer registration can be described in five central processes—*1) identification*: For a clear meaning of the definition and classification of each case included, the data should be standardized to facilitate data comparability; *2) collection*: For each cancer case, essential information such as patient data, tumor, and bases of diagnosis must be included; *3) coding*: The standardization of the nomenclature and the coding for each cancer case should provide an enabled database for comparison between different geographic areas and ease-of-analysis; *4) capture*: Due to a large amount of processed information in a cancer registry, it is recommended to use a data-processing program in order to capture data and to store information, and *5) analysis and report*: The analysis of the data in registries should periodically provide information on the cancer burden in a specific population. The report should include background information on the registry, registration procedures, catchment population, degree of data completeness and validity, methods of analysis, and findings (**Figure 1**) [16].

The statistical information produced by cancer registries could be used in different fields, including the following—etiological investigation; primary prevention (evalu-ation of cancer-control programs); secondary prevention (evaluation and monitor-ing of screening and early-detection programs), and tertiary prevention (survival analysis) and service planning, in a manner that benefits individuals as well as society as a whole [15].

2.1 Types of cancer registries

According to WHO, we could describe three different types of cancer registries—pathology-based; hospital-based, and population-based. The roles of the three types

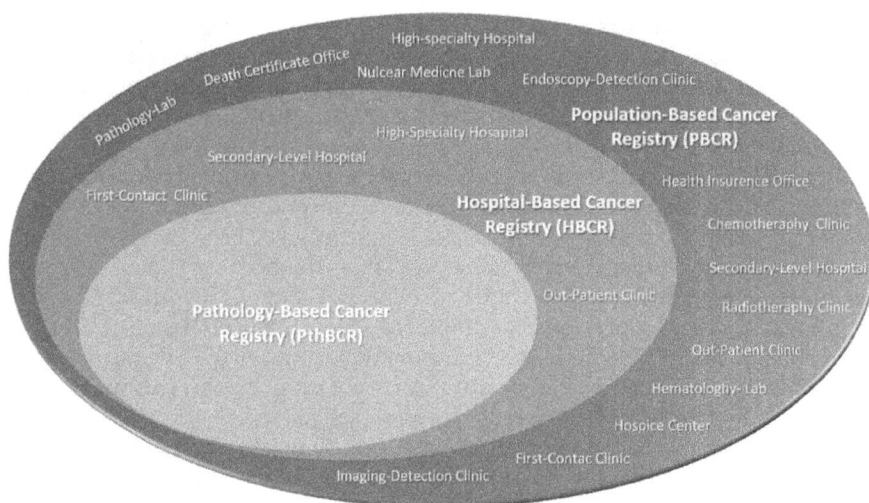

Figure 1.
Cancer registries coverage.

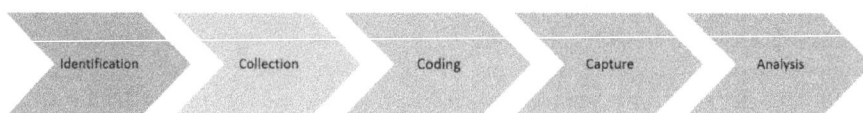

Figure 2.
Cancer registration process.

of registries are different and complementary. The first two types serve important administrative and clinical functions, but only the population-based registry provides an unbiased profile of the present cancer burden and how it changes over time. Thus, population-based cancer registries (PBCR) play a unique role in planning and evaluating population-based cancer-control actions aimed at reducing the cancer burden. Thus, PBCR is considered the gold standard, (**Figure 2**) [14]. These registries are described briefly as follows:

a. ***Pathology-based Cancer Registry (PthBCR)***. It collects information on neoplasms of *in situ* and malignant behavior from one or more pathology laboratories. Pathological data represents a potentially excellent source of case ascertainment and offers the prospect of increasing the validity of diagnosis and the accuracy of the information recorded on morphology. However, the information from PthBCR is utilized mainly for administrative laboratory purposes and represents an incomplete and skewed cancer profile, which is essentially determined by the types of tissues that the laboratory can process. Consequently, that reliance by a cancer registry on pathology data alone may lead to the loss of detail on the subsite, the registration of rare tumors, and the failure to identify cases of recurrence.

b. ***Hospital-based Cancer Registry (HBCR)***. It collects information on patients with cancer treated at one or more hospitals. The main purpose of such registries is to contribute to the care of patients by providing readily accessible information on subjects with cancer regarding the treatment they receive and the outcome. Information from HBCR is employed mainly for administrative purposes, for reviewing clinical performance, and for prioritizing hospital resources. In addition, HBCR facilitates the monitoring of health programs and allows for the detection of the patterns or frequencies of different types of cancer treated in the hospital, as well as the monitoring of the outcomes of treatment, survival rates, quality of life, and adverse treatment effects, and also supply a convenient source of patients for clinical and epidemiological studies. Information sources for HBCR include out-patient clinics, anatomopathology laboratories, hematology laboratories, nuclear medicine laboratories, autopsy and death-certificate offices, and departments of surgery, oncology, radiotherapy, chemotherapy, imaging, endoscopy, etc. HBCR provides an incomplete and skewed cancer profile because they are determined by the population treated at a specific medical center, clinic, or hospital.

c. **Population-based Cancer Registry (PBCR)**. These registries are concerned with collecting data on all new cases of cancer occurring in a well-defined population, and with being able to distinguish between residents of the area and those from outside the area. The key feature of the PCBR is the use of multiple sources of information on cancer cases. Information sources for PBCR are public and private—hospitals; cancer centers; medical offices; out-patient clinics; anatomopathology laboratories; hospice centers; hematology laboratories; nuclear medicine laboratories; imaging detection clinics; endoscopy detection clinics; chemotherapy and radiotherapy clinics; civil registry offices (death certificates); and health insurance offices. Hence, this strategy in PBCR facilitates the identification of as many as possible of cases diagnosed among the residents of the area defined by the registry. This procedure permits the identification of the same cancer case from different sources. This is regardless of whether the information on the same cases is received from several sources; indeed, this feature comprises a quality control that may be employed to evaluate success in case finding, as long as duplicate registries are avoided.

PBCR provides a more reliable cancer profile for estimating population indicators; therefore, these registries play an important role in cancer epidemiology, permitting the estimation of incidence rates by tumor location, age, gender, and other factors. Through patient tracking, it is possible to estimate cancer survival, which provides a useful indicator of this disease in the community. This method is also an affordable and efficient resource for enrolling cases for intervention and for cohort and case–control studies. Additionally, PBCR can identify geographical and temporal changes by means of the estimation of trends [15].

Additionally, the expanded role of PBCR in health systems includes the following—a) assessing differences in cancer incidence and mortality in order to address inequality in cancer prevention and care utilizing the assessment of variations in cancer frequency between different geographic areas, according to the ethnic origin, occupation, and sociodemographic status; b) monitoring the effect of primary cancer-prevention campaigns by assessing trends in cancer frequency; c) monitoring the effectiveness of cancer treatment and that of screening programs; d) planning the future needs of cancer services employing projections of cancer frequency with assumed trends in risk factors and intervention.

2.2 Procedures and quality control

In cancer registration, the quality of the data is more important than the quantity, especially for certain features and due to the large number of data produced every day. In general, medical databases possess heterogeneity, but in particular, cancer is a complex and heterogeneous disease, with hundreds of histological and biological subtypes, while on the other hand, it affects a wide range of ages, from those of children to the elderly and involves the complexity of biological variation by ethnicity. Thus, the quality-controlled data produced by the cancer registry are valued as far more effective.

Collecting information in cancer registration can be active or passive; in general, the majority of registries utilize a combination of both methods. The active procedure involves visiting the sources of information, reviewing these, and abstracting the information into a special format by the cancer-registry staff, while the passive procedure relies upon routine notifications from hospitals, laboratories, and death records; thus, the registry may periodically receive abstracts, notifications, or databases [8, 16].

Depending on utility, purpose, logistics, and budget, the cancer registry must collect essential information on the patients, the tumor, the source, and additional information. It is recommendable that each domain contains the following information in as complete a form as possible; *1) Patient information*: Full name, age, gender, birthplace, address, identification number (if applicable, because some countries use a unique ID number), and ethnic group; *2) Tumor information*: Incidence date, primary tumor site (topography), laterality (if applicable), morphology, behavior, the base of diagnosis, and date of death (if applicable); *3) Information source*: Hospital, clinic, and laboratory name or number (the place where the cancer was diagnosed), and *4) Other details*: It is recommended that these be collected, depending on the capacity and applicability of the registry, such as the following—biomarkers; genomic information; disease stages; treatment information (surgery, radiation, chemotherapy, hormone therapy, and immunotherapy), and outcomes such as vital status (alive, dead, or lost to follow-up) [14, 17].

Patient Information: Identification items such as name, gender, and date of birth are important to avoid multiple registrations of the same patient or the tumor, in order to obtain follow-up data and record linkage. The patient's address is essential for establishing residence status. Data on ethnicity is important in populations containing diverse ethnic groups.

Tumor Information: Incidence date is primarily the date of the first histological or cytological confirmations of the malignancy, as this is a definite, consistent, and reliable point in time that can be verified from records. If this information is not available, the date should be taken of the first diagnosis by the physician, or the date of the first pathological report, or the date of death, if no information is available other than that the patient died or if the malignancy is discovered at autopsy.

Since cancer is not a single disease, but instead a complex and heterogeneous one with hundreds of histological and biological subtypes, it is thus recommended that the cancer registry use the International Classification of Diseases for Oncology (ICD-O) to code the tumor. The ICD-O is a multi-axial classification of topography (site of primary tumor), morphology (histological type), behavior (benign, borderline, *in situ*, malignant), grading (differentiation), and bases of diagnosis (information on how the tumor was diagnosed, by means of a clinical history only, or by exploratory surgery, laboratory, biomarkers, autopsy, imaging (X-ray, ultrasound, etc.), or anatomopathologically). The topography of the tumor is the most important data item recorded and provides the main basis for the tabulation of registry data.

Information Source: For purposes of future checking, it is important for the registry to collect data on the sources of the cancer case-finding, for instance, name of the physician, hospital, laboratory, biopsy number, etc. This additional information will help to trace the medical records of the patients.

Recommendations. a) New record: For new cancer cases, it is recommendable to use a unique registration number for each patient. If the patient has more than one primary tumor, a different number is given to each tumor in order to facilitate the consultation, operation, management, and analysis. One key challenge is to store the patient's identifiable data, which is mandatory for safeguarding the patient's privacy; for each patient, personal information data, including name and national identification number (ID), and personal sensitive data such as addresses, phone number, and gender, must be unidentified. All of the databases should contain a security framework to provide authentication, authorization, and to audit the systems. *b) Multiple tumors*: If there are several records for the same patient, the most appropriate primary tumor by topography, morphology, and incidence date must be determined. The second primary tumor is defined as a new record on an individual who has already been recorded. *c) Duplicate tumor*: When matching by name, allowance must be made for errors in spelling (the phonetic spelling of names or errors due to the illegibility of hospital records). The strategy is to match first by name, then by age, gender, address, and diagnosis, to ensure that it is a real duplicate. If there is no match, it is a new patient who should be registered as a new record [14, 16].

Cancer registration is not only a system for the classification and the coding of neoplasms. It also requires a clear definition of what constitutes a cancer case, the definition of the date of incidence, and the rules for dealing with multiple primary cancers, including the need to differentiate between a new case of primary cancer and the extension, recurrence, or metastasis of an existing one. Therefore, trained personnel and adherence to international standards for registering cancer cases are necessary.

Because data collection by the different registries around the world may vary according to local needs and the availability of information, the value of cancer-registry information depends on producing reliable and comparable national and international cancer data; hence, cancer registry must adopt and follow rules for coding, data-quality standards, and procedures. The International Association of Cancer Registry (IACR), the International Agency for Research on Cancer (IARC), and the Global Initiative for Cancer Registry (GIRC) have produced guidelines and recommendations regarding the data items collected [14, 18].

The Global Initiative for Cancer Registry Development (GICR) was launched and is coordinated by IARC, with its main purpose being to support local planning and reduce the cancer-registration disparities between low- and middle-income countries by building local and sustainable infrastructure through regional centers of expertise-denominated IARC regional hubs. Over the last few years, IARC has established regional hubs for cancer registration in Africa, Asia, and Latin America. These hubs provide a set of local activities in a given country for increasing data quality, coverage, and utility in terms of cancer-control proposes, through technical guidance, training, advocacy, data collection, analysis, and promoting cancer research by identifying top-ics of common interest to the community that directly contribute to cancer control, thus fostering collaborative cancer research across countries [14].

According to IARC, cancer registries should be able to furnish some objective indication of the quality described in the following four dimensions—*a) Comparability*: Because one of the main topics of cancer registries is the comparison of statistical results, the standardization is required of practices concerning the classification and coding of new cases and regarding consistency in definitions of incidence, such as rules for the recording and reporting of multiple primary cancers occurring in the same patient. WHO published the International Classification Diseases of Oncology (ICD-O) as a standard for classifying and coding cancer as follows; *b) Exhaustivity*: It defines the degree of the population covered by the registry; in particular, PBCR should, by definition, register every single case that occurs in its catchment population. On the other hand, for the case ascertainment, there are certain methods to determine the degree of completeness of registration, such as comparison with death certificates and cancer-registry records; *c) Validity*: It defines the accuracy of the work of the staff with the accuracy of recorded data that are greatly enhanced by consistency checks carried out at the time of data entry. Data validity can be assessed in several ways, such as the proportion of cases with microscopic verification of diagnosis, a very useful index, because it may represent the incompleteness of data collection, and such as re-abstracting and re-coding a sample of cases to assess validity data. *d) Opportunity*: It defines the trade-off between data timeliness and the extent to which the data are complete for reporting. Timeliness depends on the time during which the registry can collect, process, and report complete and accurate data. Methods such as a delay model estimate the undercount at the time of reporting, which gives an indication of the degree of completeness relative to other registries [19, 20].

2.3 Prevention and control

Accurate information on cancer burden is important in establishing priorities and targeting cancer-control activities. PBCR forms an essential part of rationale programs of cancer control. The annual number of incident cancer cases (new cases) provides an indication of the resources needed for primary treatment, and the number of prevalent cancer cases (new and old cases) describes how many individuals are in need of regular long-term follow-up [15]. Therefore, cancer-registry data can be utilized in a wide variety of areas of cancer control, ranging from etiological research through primary prevention, health-care planning, and patient care. Consequently, prevention, screening, and early detection entertain overlapping goals—either that of avoiding cancer altogether or treating it when the odds of success are at their highest. Thus, prevention can be primary when avoiding the effective contact of a carcinogenic agent with a susceptible target person. Prevention is secondary when stopping the disease from the beginning by the detection of a precursor lesion at an individual patient's check-up, or through population screening, while it is tertiary when it includes strategies to promote the early detection of second primary cancers, as well as follow-up and treatment-related complications in cancer survivors.

a. *Primary prevention.* Prevention is implemented in two ways—a) by the avoidance, interruption, or abatement of carcinogenic exposure, and b) by vaccination, such as that of hepatitis B virus (HBV) or papillomavirus (VPH) or by dietary chemoprevention (increasing vegetable intake). Hence, cancer registries can play an important role in monitoring and evaluating the effectiveness of primary prevention. For instance, trends in the incidence of cancer can be related to changes over time in exposure to cancer risk factors. Therefore, public-health initiatives such as reducing smoking, curbing obesity, and improving cancer screening and vaccination rates could be furthered by targeting messages to the person at risk of cancer or those with susceptibility to cancer, based on cancer-registry information. Cancer-registry information can also be employed for monitoring occupational groups of individuals at risk for exposure to various carcinogens or even to promote health-care education that influences behavior or social influences or directly on patients [15, 21].

b. *Secondary prevention*. Prevention by screening or early detection involves the use of tests to detect cancer before the appearance of signs or symptoms. The value of early detection lies in the possibility of detecting cancer when it is still localized and more easily curable. Cancer registries can play an important role in the evaluation and monitoring of screening programs aimed at detecting preinvasive conditions; in some cases, the disease can be detected in a premalignant state, for instance, dysplasia of the cervix or stomach, and adenomas of the colon. Cancer-registry information has been used in routine data-based studies to examine trends in disease rate in relation to screening frequencies within a population and to compare disease rates between different populations with the coverage offered by their screening programs. The benefits of secondary prevention include the possibility of simpler and less expensive treatment, as well as less pain and disability [15, 22].

c. *Tertiary prevention*. Tertiary prevention includes the ongoing surveillance, care, and rehabilitation of patients with cancer, the early detection of second primary malignancies, and other treatment-related complications in cancer survivors. Tertiary prevention should reduce risk factors for second malignancies and for other long-term complications. Although more persons are living longer after an initial diagnosis of cancer, environmental and lifestyle risk factors, treatment modalities, and the underlying genetic basis of many cancers predispose survivors to develop second primary malignancies. Other complications that have recently become more evident are long-term adverse effects from chemotherapy that require assessment and early management, these effects include cardiotoxicity, neuropathy, ototoxicity, renal failure, and the development of osteoporosis in women with hormone-dependent malignancies. Cancer registries can play an important role in providing survival-analysis data that are useful in the evaluation of cancer care in the area covered by the registry, in that all cancer cases will be included regardless of the type of treatment they may have received. Time trends in survival are useful to assess the extent to which advances in treatment have exerted an effect on the population. Cancer survival is a key index of the overall effectiveness of health services in the management of patients. Differences in survival have prompted or guided cancer-control strategies [15, 23].

2.4 From the manual to the bioinformatics era

The approach of recording information on all cancer cases in defined communities dates from the first half of the twentieth century, and there has been a steady growth in the number of cancer registries. Prior to past decades, data from tumors and patients were collated via a manual process; consequently, this led to a limited variety, slow procedure, and low accuracy. In manual cancer registries, the incoming documents were checked against an index, this index generally with information recorded on cards and arranged alphabetically by name. Each index card would contain the complete case information. With the beginning of computer technology and the increasing number of computerized data sources for cancer registries, the traditional operation changed, moving from paper to digital-data sources, and with the introduction of electronic medical records, it currently generates gigabytes of information per day [16, 18].

Perhaps the biggest change and the most relevant innovation in health-care data is related to information technology (IT), which is a multidisciplinary area that combines software bioengineering, electronics, and computer science. These technological advances can also improve cancer registration by integrating electronic medical records, linkage with data sources, digital monitoring, and new diagnostic technologies, which at present produce an unprecedented quantity and diversity of routine electronic data. Cancer-registry databases are often combined with other electronic health records, such as laboratory results, vital signs (imaging files, radiography), physician notes, etc., because patients may receive cancer care at multiple services within a clinic or hospital, both public or private, within a region or geographic area. Consequently, the amount of data collected and stored digitally is growing exponentially, and it is critical for the adoption of new IT is critical to attend to this large amount of data in order to acquire a more comprehensive and accurate picture of the cancer burden [24].

Particularly, the cancer-registration database should provide several functionalities, such as patients' information, medical records, analyses, and reports. WHO launched CanReg software, an open-source tool developed by IARC especially designed to input, store, check, and analyze population-based cancer-registry data. CanReg software is updated with checks on consistency according to the international guidelines as follows—age-incidence-birth place; age-site-histology; site-histology; behavior-site; behavior-histology; and basis of diagnosis-histology. CanReg5 is available in the Chinese, English, French, Portuguese, Russian, and Spanish languages and can be downloaded free of charge from the International Association of Cancer Registries (IARC) [14].

Advancing data-processing technologies and bioinformatics are of paramount importance in understanding Big Data in cancer registration. Bioinformatics uses advanced mathematical algorithms and technological platforms to store and transform data into an interpretable format. Recently, there has been an increased usage of virtual repositories or "data clouds" to link and improve access; additionally, the cognitive computing of "artificial intelligence" and machine learning are gaining in popularity [25]. The use of new cutting-edge disciplines to generate and analyze data is a trend that has evolved between traditional medicine and precision medicine.

a. *Big Data*: Usually, this has been used to develop systems to organize and compile large-scale datasets that cannot be captured, managed, or processed by common software tools. Currently, Big Data is characterized by the *5V* as follows—*1) volume*: Big Data is large in size, containing many data records of multiple subjects; these include diagnostic work-ups such as clinical, radiological, and pathological and treatment data, and surgery, systematic therapy, radiotherapy, response, and complications; *2) variety*: Big Data comprises an enormous variability in data types and include several given data types such as weight, laboratory results, etc. Many different data types enrich the quality, and usefulness and challenges regarding whether their heterogeneity warrants standardization; *3) velocity*: Big Data possesses two velocity aspects—a) to create at an increasingly high speed, and b) to be computed relatively rapidly;

4) *veracity*: Incorrect data values or missing data undermine the ability to draw acute statistical conclusions on the distribution of values and the relationship between data elements, and 5) *value:* Setting up a data infrastructure to collect and interpret data is only worthwhile if it enables the generation of data-derived conclusions or measurements based on accurate data that can truly lead to measurable improvements or impacts on cancer healthcare [26, 27]. However, the potential of Big Data remains to be discovered for cancer registration, especially in LMIC, because medical Big-Data mining continues to face challenges, mainly due to that in these countries the hospital electronic medical-records system is missing or is poor in openness, scalability, and budget.

b. *Data Mining:* This can search for potentially valuable knowledge from a large amount of data, mainly divided into data preparation, data mining, and the expression and analysis of results, processed with methods in terms of the structure, storage, design, management, and application of the database. The purpose of the emergence of data-mining technology is not to replace traditional statistical-analysis technology but is the extension of the statistical-analysis methodology. Data-mining methods can be divided into the following two categories that can be applied in cancer registration—descriptive and predictive. Descriptive patterns characterize the general nature of data, including association analysis and cluster analysis, while predictive patterns are summarized on current data, including classification and regression [27].

c. *Artificial Intelligence*: This paradigm represents a novel frontier and innovative tools for cancer control. Current epidemiological research in conjunction with cutting-edge informatics technologies produces data mining and artificial intelligence (AI). Artificial intelligence is conventionally defined as the ability of a computer system to perform acts of problem solving, reasoning, and learning, and, among all of the latter, independent learning is the most important ability, as it mitigates the need for human intervention to continually enhance the performance of the system for it to work more efficiently with increased reliability and timeliness [28, 29].

3. Conclusion

Given the diversity of cancers in different geographic areas, it is necessary to base cancer-control activities on customized cancer profiles obtained through cancer registration.

Global figures of the burden of cancer across the different geographic areas are made possible by cancer-registry data. The most efficient method for addressing the cancer challenge is by means of the development and implantation of a cancer-control plan whose core indicator is the cancer registry.

Cancer-registry statistical results could be used in different fields. These include etiological investigation, primary prevention (evaluation of cancer-control programs to avoid carcinogenic exposure and vaccination), secondary prevention (evaluation and monitoring of screening and early-detection programs), and tertiary prevention (evaluation of care and rehabilitation in cancer survivor patients, the impact of changes over time, and survival analysis), for the benefit of individuals as well as of society as a whole.

The technological revolution of recent years is an unprecedented event that has impacted the health-care field, and consequently, cancer registration.

Acknowledgements

The author wishes to express her gratitude to the Merida Population-Based Cancer Registry.

Conflict of interest

The author declares no potential conflict of interest.

Author details

Yelda A. Leal
Institutional Center for Training and Cancer Registry, High Specialty Medical Unit (UMAE), Mexican Social Security Institute (IMSS), Merida, Yucatan, Mexico

*Address all correspondence to: yelda_leal03@yahoo.com.mx; yelda.leal@imss.gob.mx

IntechOpen

References

[1] Ghebreyesus TA. Acting on NCDs: Counting the cost. Lancet. 2018; **391**(10134):1973-1974

[2] WHO. Global Action Plan for the Prevention and Control of NonCommunicable Diseases 2013-2020. Geneva, Switzerland: World Health Organization; 2013. p. 91

[3] Bray F, Ferlay J, Soerjomataram I, Siegel RL, Torre LA, Jemal A. Global cancer statistics 2018: GLOBOCAN estimates of incidence and mortality worldwide for 36 cancers in 185 countries. CA: a Cancer Journal for Clinicians. 2018;**68**(6):394-424

[4] WHO. Cancer prevention and control in the context of an integrated approach. In: WHO, editor. The Seventieth World Health Assembly. Geneva, Switzerland: WHO; 2017. p. 6

[5] WHO. Draft, Comprehensive Global Monitoring Framework and Targets for the Prevention and Control of NCDs. Geneva, Switzerland: WHO; 2013. p. 9

[6] Pineros M, Abriata MG, Mery L, Bray F. Cancer registration for cancer control in Latin America: A status and progress report. Revista Panamericana de Salud Pública. 2017;**41**:e2

[7] Brucher BL, Jamall IS. Epistemology of the origin of cancer: A new paradigm. BMC Cancer. 2014;**14**:331

[8] Leal YA, Fernández-Garrote LM, Mohar-Betancourt A, Meneses-García A. The importance of registries in cancer control. Salud Pública de México. 2016;**58**(2):309-316

[9] Katzke VA, Kaaks R, Kuhn T. Lifestyle and cancer risk. Cancer Journal. 2015;**21**(2):104-110

[10] Bray F, Jemal A, Grey N, Ferlay J, Forman D. Global cancer transitions according to the Human Development Index (2008-2030): A population-based study. The Lancet Oncology. 2012; **13**(8):790-801

[11] Cogliano VJ, Baan R, Straif K, Grosse Y, Lauby-Secretan B, El Ghissassi F, et al. Preventable exposures associated with human cancers. Journal of the National Cancer Institute. 2011; **103**(24):1827-1839

[12] Prager GW, Braga S, Bystricky B, Qvortrup C, Criscitiello C, Esin E, et al. Global cancer control: Responding to the growing burden, rising costs and inequalities in access. ESMO Open. 2018;**3**(2):e000285

[13] de Martel C, Georges D, Bray F, Ferlay J, Clifford GM. Global burden of cancer attributable to infections in 2018: A worldwide incidence analysis. The Lancet Global Health. 2020;**8**(2): e180-ee90

[14] Bray F, Znaor A, Cueva P, Korir A, Rajaraman S, Ullrich A, et al. Planing and Developing Population-Based Cancer Registration in Low- and Middle-Income Settings. Lyon, France: International Agency for Research on Cancer; 2014

[15] dos Santos-Silva I. Cancer Epidemiology: Principles and Methods. Lyon, France: International Agency for Research on Cancer; 1999

[16] Jensen OP, Parkin DM, MacLennan R, Muir CS, Skeet RG. Cancer Registration: Principles and Merthods. Lyon, France: International Agency for Research on Cancer; 1991

[17] Curado MP, Voti L, Sortino-Rachou AM. Cancer registration data and quality indicators in low and middle income countries: Their interpretation and potential use for the improvement of cancer care. Cancer Causes & Control. 2009;**20**(5):751-756

[18] Parkin DM. The evolution of the population-based cancer registry. Nature Reviews. Cancer. 2006;**6**(8):603-612

[19] Bray F, Parkin DM. Evaluation of data quality in the cancer registry: Principles and methods. Part I. Comparability, Validity and Timeliness. European Journal of Cancer. 2009; **45**(5):747-755

[20] Parkin DM, Bray F. Evaluation of data quality in the cancer registry: Principles and methods, Part II. Completeness. European Journal of Cancer. 2009;**45**(5):756-764

[21] Adami HO, Day NE, Trichopoulos D, Willett WC. Primary and secondary prevention in the reduction of cancer morbidity and mortality. European Journal of Cancer. 2001;**37**(Suppl 8): S118-S127

[22] Eddy DM. Secondary prevention of cancer: An overview. Bulletin of the World Health Organization. 1986; **64**(3):421-429

[23] Mahon SM. Tertiary prevention: Implications for improving the quality of life of long-term survivors of cancer. Seminars in Oncology Nursing. 2005; **21**(4):260-270

[24] Schlick CJR, Castle JP, Bentrem DJ. Utilizing big data in cancer care. Surgical Oncology Clinics of North America. 2018;**27**(4):641-652

[25] Tsai CJ, Riaz N, Gómez SL. Big Data in cancer research: Real-world resources for precision oncology to improve cancer care delivery. Seminars in Radiation Oncology. 2019;**29**(4):306-310

[26] Willems SM, Abeln S, Feenstra KA, de Bree R, van der Poel EF, Baatenburg de Jong RJ, et al. The potential use of big data in oncology. Oral Oncology. 2019; **98**:8-12

[27] Yang J, Li Y, Liu Q, Li L, Feng A, Wang T, et al. Brief introduction of medical database and data mining technology in Big Bata era. Journal of Evidence-Based Medicine. 2020;**13**(1): 57-69

[28] Yu C, Helwig EJ. The role of AI technology in prediction, diagnosis and treatment of colorectal cancer. Artificial Intelligence Review. 2021. https://doi. org/10.1007/s10462-021-10034-y

[29] Arora A. Conceptualising artificial intelligence as a digital healthcare innovation: An introductory review. Medical Devices (Auckl). 2020; **13**:223-230

Chapter 7

Dotting the "i" of Interoperability in FAIR Cancer-Registry Data Sets

Nicholas Nicholson, Francesco Giusti, Luciana Neamtiu,
Giorgia Randi, Tadeusz Dyba, Manola Bettio,
Raquel Negrao Carvalho, Nadya Dimitrova,
Manuela Flego and Carmen Martos

Abstract

To conform to FAIR principles, data should be findable, accessible, interoperable, and reusable. Whereas tools exist for making data findable and accessible, interoperability is not straightforward and can limit data reusability. Most interoperability-based solutions address semantic description and metadata linkage, but these alone are not sufficient for the requirements of inter-comparison of population-based cancer data, where strict adherence to data-rules is of paramount importance. Ontologies, and more importantly their formalism in description logics, can play a key role in the automation of data-harmonization processes predominantly via the formalization of the data validation rules within the data-domain model. This in turn leads to a potential quality metric allowing users or agents to determine the limitations in the interpretation and comparability of the data. An approach is described for cancer-registry data with practical examples of how the validation rules can be modeled with description logic. Conformance of data to the rules can be quantified to provide metrics for several quality dimensions. Integrating these with metrics derived for other quality dimensions using tools such as data-shape languages and data-completion tests builds up a data-quality context to serve as an additional component in the FAIR digital object to support interoperability in the wider sense.

Keywords: cancer registries, data interoperability, ontologies, description logics data harmonization, data validation, data quality, FAIR data

1. Introduction

Comparison of cancer indicators across different regions and countries is important to understand the effectiveness of cancer prevention and control measures. Considerable care has to be taken however to ensure that the data are indeed comparable and have the necessary level of quality not to result in the production of biased or misleading statistics. Centralized processes to ensure comparability of data are costly in terms of time and resources and should ideally be supported with efficient and effective automated tools. The goal towards the eventual federation of such processes requires the means of formally ascertaining the level of the quality of the underlying data.

1.1 Population-based cancer registries

Population-based cancer registries (CRs) are information systems designed for the collection, storage, and management of data on cancer patients. They collate information on all cancer cases occurring in a defined population and play a critical role in the planning and evaluation of cancer control activities at population level (particularly via trends in incidence, mortality, prevalence, and survival), as well as in identifying good practices of patient care [1, 2]. They also provide the means for evaluating the effectiveness of screening programs and contribute actively to cancer epidemiological research.

CRs may be nationally based, covering the entire country (such as in Europe for Finland, Sweden, and Slovenia), or regionally based (such as in France, Italy, and Spain). Whereas regional CRs may provide total coverage of the country, in some cases they only provide partial coverage and estimations based on the partial coverage are used to provide national statistics. The production of reliable statistics is directly dependent on the quality of the underlying CR data.

1.2 CR data collection and cleaning process

The data collected by a CR are in accordance with the purpose for which the registry has been established, dependent on the available information and resources. Nevertheless, the accent is on the quality of the data rather than on the quantity [3]. Whereas the initial focus was on monitoring cancer incidence and the trends over time, many registries now collect patient follow-up details in order to compute survival.

CRs need to register all cancers diagnosed in a defined area and have consequently to access multiple data sources, including hospital discharge and outpatient records, pathology laboratory results, oncology/radiotherapy/clinical hematology records and death certificates. The combination of such sources is the cornerstone of the data collection process [4]. Additional data sources include screening programs, communications from general practitioners, drug prescriptions, and insurance reimbursement claims.

Sets of rules and linkage routines are normally used to create provisional incidence records, which are then verified within a few months to confirm or discard cases [5]. Once the incidence data set has been consolidated, the data are thereafter cleaned according to specific data-cleaning rules. Additional to the local CR procedures, wider standards for data collection, coding, reporting, and validation are required to facilitate data interoperability. Such standards are generally defined and agreed at national or transnational level, especially in relation to the data comprising the base denominator or the common data set.

1.3 Importance of CR data harmonization

Within the last couple of decades, CR data have improved dramatically in quality and quantity, due largely to technological advances and the improved means for reliable record linkage [6, 7]. Owing to the fact that CRs collect and integrate data from very heterogeneous multiple information sources, a process of data harmonization is required both preceding and following linkage according to national and internationally accepted procedures. This process of harmonization has been defined as "all efforts to combine data from different sources and provide users with a comparable view of data from different studies" [8] and is a critical element for accurate and meaningful inter-comparison of CR data. It is also extremely important for the correct usage of anonymized or aggregated CR data in secondary-data analyses [9].

An example of the importance of CR data harmonization relates to the implementation of the 1995 European Network of Cancer Registries' (ENCR) recommendations for the coding of bladder tumors in the Scottish CRs in the year 2000. After the introduction of the recommendations, bladder tumor incidence rates halved [10] and became similar to those of other registries following the same rules. Notwithstanding such changes in coding, it always remains possible to calculate rates with the previous rules in order to assess time trends.

1.4 CR associations and networks

In the US, the North American Association of Central Cancer Registries (NAACR) develops and promotes uniform data standards for cancer registration. These standardization efforts are of direct importance to the North American Surveillance, Epidemiology, and End Results (SEER) program [11] involving twenty-one North American CRs covering more than one third of the U.S. population.

Within Europe, the standardization efforts of the ENCR, comprising over 150 individual registries, are similarly of importance to the European Cancer Information System (ECIS) [12]. The International Association of Cancer Registries (IACR), the International Agency for Research on Cancer (IARC), the European Commission, and ENCR have all played an essential role in European CR harmonization.

The harmonization efforts ultimately benefit endeavors to compare cancer statistics at the global level [13, 14]. Data harmonization for inter-comparison purposes is generally achieved via the specification of common data sets in which the ranges and interdependencies of a core set of variables are defined by an agreed set of specific rules. The harmonization process is time consuming and requires consultation and agreement across a wide range of stakeholders, especially when the common data set serves multiple purposes. An example of a common data set comprising some fifty data variables and the rules specifying the variable values/ranges and the inter-variable relationships is provided in [15]. The ENCR common data set includes variables related to the patient, the tumor (including stage), treatment, and follow-up.

Owing to the need to ensure a high and consistent level of quality and harmonization, the CR common data sets are currently collected and processed centrally. Whereas centralized processes help control and ensure consistency, they add extra time delays in making the data available – not least from the overheads occasioned by increasingly stricter data-protection paradigms. Data cleaning and harmonization for CR inter-comparison purposes could be made more efficient by devolving the centralized processes to the local level – so long as consistency and data quality can be assured. Conformance of CR data to the FAIR data principles is key to realizing this aim.

1.5 FAIR data principles

The four principles of FAIR data, encompassed in their felicitously named acronym, underlie the need for data to be: findable, accessible, interoperable, and reusable [16], also at a machine-readable and inferable level. The meaning of each term is elaborated by a set of three or four qualifying elements. The challenges to

FAIR data principle	Questions to address	Possible means for addressing the needs
Findable	Do the data exist and where exactly?	Data catalogs and inter-linkage of catalogs, with relevant search functions; registration of the data under unique identifiers; persistent links and identifiers; searchable metadata; appropriate synonym lists for search terms
Accessible	Is authorization needed to access the data? How can the data be accessed physically?	Data access and user identification controls; authorization request interfaces; application programing interfaces; data extraction scripts; file format metadata; identification of relevant application tools
Interoperable	Can the data be integrated/combined fully/partially with another data set? Can the data be loaded from different applications? Are the data properly comparable with other data? What is the context of the data? How do the variables inter-relate? What are the measurement units of the variables? How can the measurement units be mapped to similar terms in another data set measured in different units?	Metadata descriptions of data variables; linkage of metadata terms to standard data dictionaries; mapping systems; knowledge organization systems; data quality contexts
Reusable	Does the data set contain limitations/disclaimers/assumptions? Are there data restrictions/licenses? Can the data be used for other purposes? Will the data still be accessible at a future date? May the data change over time?	Contextual and provenance metadata; data-usage licenses; data persistence mechanisms; data-maintenance policies

Table 1.
Challenges involved in making data FAIR, some of the questions that have to be addressed, and possible mechanisms for addressing them.

making data FAIR, in terms of the questions that have to be addressed, and some of the mechanisms towards meeting those challenges are summarized in **Table 1**.

The foundations of FAIR were in fact laid down in several earlier initiatives [17] and the EU is actively supporting activities to progress the underlying concepts. Interoperability is arguably the most challenging of the four FAIR data principles outside of access to personalized data and is discussed further in Section 2. In relation to findable data, health data providers in many countries have started to create data portals and data catalogs.

Whereas a number of international CR portals provide access to anonymized and aggregated CR data sets [11, 12], it is not usually possible to provide secure access to record-level data through automated protocols due to the sensitive nature of health data, although SEER does provide an example of a way to access cancer data following a set of specific conditions. The challenges to CR data accessibility as far as record-level data are concerned are in fact less technical than administrative in view of the legal aspects of data-protection laws. Indeed, they are generic to all data where identification of a person is possible and, even with anonymized data sets, care has to be taken to ensure that persons cannot be re-identified using other data sources. Steps are being taken in the EU, where the data-protection laws are amongst the strictest in the world, to address mechanisms to facilitate authorized access to health data.

Reusability for CR data mainly refers to their use for secondary-data purposes and hinges on accurate and comprehensive description of the data in both the contextual and semantic sense. In this regard, there is a close relationship with the principle of semantic interoperability (c.f. Section 2.1) – if the data are comprehensively described, the possibility for data reuse is greatly assisted. The latter may be appreciated to some extent by considering SEER data, which are well described in terms of metadata and draw from data adhering to the NACCR data standards. SEER data have consequently led to hundreds of scientific publications on cancer epidemiology. In contrast, the health data environment in Europe is extremely fragmented, but recent initiatives on data reuse are described in [18], including national initiatives in Finland, France, Portugal, and Italy. Within the EU as a whole, the first preparatory steps have been undertaken to create a European Health Data Space (EHDS) [19] for facilitating primary and secondary reuse of health data.

2. Data interoperability

The three qualifying elements defined under FAIR's interoperability principle [16] are in relation to knowledge representation – with particular reference to the use of formal, shared languages and vocabularies as well as linkage to other data descriptors/ metadata. Such aspects largely refer to syntactic and semantic interoperability.

2.1 Semantic interoperability

Mechanisms to address semantic interoperability include metadata schemas drawing on standard data dictionaries and thesauri, metadata catalogs (e.g. Data Catalog Vocabulary, DCAT [20]), metadata registries (e.g., ISO/IEC 11179 metadata registry standard [21]), knowledge organization systems (e.g. Simple Knowledge Organization System – SKOS [22]), linked open data (LOD) or any combination of these. Such mechanisms can be incorporated into frameworks and architectures designed for the purposes of supporting FAIR data processes.

A non-exclusive list of FAIR-supporting infrastructures include: beacons [23, 24], used primarily for discovering and sharing of genomic data; a federated semantic metadata registry framework [25], which also provides a potential model for population-based patient registries including CRs [26]; the MOLGENIS data platform for data sharing [27]; the Apache Atlas data governance and metadata framework [28]; the European Open Science Cloud (EOSC) interoperability framework [29]; and the FAIR digital object framework [30]. The way in which the FAIR digital object concept is able to support data interoperability, particularly with reference to EOSC, has been discussed in [31].

The main challenges to semantic interoperability lie in the interlinkage, mapping, and maintenance of metadata between different standards and systems. The availability of standard dictionaries and ontologies together with knowledge organization systems such as SKOS allow data providers to describe their record-level metadata variables in ways meaningful for data users to combine data sets from different data sources. The fact that these standard resources are available in machine-readable ways opens up the possibility for automation of the data-linkage process by intelligent agents, especially when used in conjunction with data registration and cataloging systems.

As important as the semantic context of data is, it does not fulfill all the requirements to make data interoperable. According to the Data Interoperability Standards

Consortium [32], data interoperability concerns "the ability of systems and services that create, exchange and consume data to have clear, shared expectations for the contents, context and meaning of that data."

Whereas semantic definitions and linkages of metadata can help describe the context and meaning of data, they cannot per se vouch for the quality of the data. Data quality is of prime importance for CRs whose data are compared between regions and countries for epidemiological purposes or for gauging the effectiveness of cancer healthcare policy initiatives.

2.2 Data quality

Without having some information regarding the quality and veracity of the data sets to be combined, any assumptions drawn from the data integration will at best be speculative. The FAIR data principles do not explicitly address such aspects, apart from in the sense that the usefulness of the data is somehow determinable by the user [33]. One of the qualifying elements under the reusable principle however does require that (meta)data meet domain-relevant community standards, of which quality could arguably form a part, and acknowledgement is given to the critical importance of the quality dimension as identified in the initiatives on which FAIR builds [17].

Various ways for defining data quality have been propounded, particularly in relation to terms of classification/categorization. The ideas build on research conducted in the 1990s, mainly in relation to total data quality management (TDQM) for business processes. An overview of this early work [34] further developed the ideas and formulated a hierarchical data-quality framework in order to addresses the contemporary needs of big data with a view to developing data-quality evaluation algorithms. The hierarchy consists of fourteen elements (with a number of associated indicators) classified under the five dimensions of: availability, usability, reliability, relevance, and presentation quality. Most of these dimensions turn out to be closely aligned with the FAIR data principles and are therefore inherent to the objectives of the FAIR digital object framework (FDOF) [30]. The FDOF provides the means of resolving the identifier associated with a FAIR digital object into sets of information relating to the features required by the FAIR data principles. Factoring out these commonalities essentially removes all but the "reliability" dimension (equating to the trustworthiness of data) in the hierarchy of [34] and one of the elements (Timeliness) under the "availability" dimension as summarized in **Table 2**.

Despite the lack of a universally agreed data-quality system, five of the resulting six elements are common to five of the six quality dimensions identified in [35], which also provides suggested metrics. The different sixth elements are "auditability" and "uniqueness" respectively. In total, the seven quality elements (which we refer to as quality dimensions in line with the terminology used in [35]) are described in **Table 3** together with the proposed means of measurement:

ISO 8000 is an international standard for managing, measuring, and improving the quality of data. Part 8 of the standard [36] (Information and data quality: Concepts and Measuring) can be used independently of the other parts and is specifically focused on providing the means for measuring the quality of data and information against scales that the standard requires the enterprise to establish. It can therefore be used as a means for auditing the data quality.

ISO 8000-8 categorizes data/information quality under: syntactic quality, semantic quality, and pragmatic quality. Syntactic quality relates to the degree in which the data/information conforms to its metadata specifications and the standard

Big data quality dimension	Big data quality element	FAIR principle
Availability	Accessibility	A
	Timeliness	—
	Authorization	A
Usability	Definition/documentation	I,R
	Credibility	R
	MetaData	F,I
Reliability	Accuracy	—
	Integrity	—
	Consistency	—
	Completeness	—
	Auditability	—
Relevance	Fitness	R
Presentation quality	Readability	A,I
	Structure	A,I

Table 2.
Cross-matrix of the quality dimensions (and associated elements) proposed for big-data quality [34] with the different FAIR principles.

Dimension	Measure	Unit of measure
Completeness	Degree in which all the essential data are provided. Can be measured at both data level (missing data records) and variable level (missing variables within a record)	Percentage/ratio (e.g. proportion of captured data against potential of 100%)
Integrity/ Validity	Degree in which data types are standardized or conform to rules and relations encapsulated in the data.	Percentage/ratio (e.g. number of non-conformant data elements missing as a ratio of number of records).
Consistency	Differences found for data entities (or their representations) that should be identical or equivalent	Number (e.g. number of differences)
Accuracy	Degree in which the real-life situation is different from its representation	Percentage (e.g. percentage of records to that pass pre-specified data-accuracy rules;
Timeliness	Degree in which the data are representative of the current situation	Time difference
Uniqueness	Redundancy of data which could otherwise be derived, leading to maintenance and consistency issues	Percentage to total of duplicates data/data variables
Auditability	Ease in which/extent to which auditors can evaluate the quality of the data	An agreed or standardized scale

Table 3.
Description and proposed units of measurement of the seven generally agreed data-quality dimensions.

requires the specification of a full set of syntactic quality rules. Semantic quality relates to the correspondence/relationships of data or information to other entities as represented in a conceptual model. The standard requires a documented conceptual model and a description of the means used for verification against the model. Pragmatic quality concerns usage-based requirements that have to be expressed as specific perspectives or dimensions not covered by the other two quality criteria. It can relate to such aspects as accessibility, completeness, security, etc. Using a standard such as ISO 8000-8 would address the issue of auditability as well as allow the means for formally specifying the other six quality dimensions and the metrics for their measurement.

2.2.1 Quality metrics of CR common data set

Regarding the CR common data set, the metrics related to variable-completeness (i.e. completeness of the common data mandatory variable set), timeliness, and uniqueness can be relatively easily defined. The common data set specifies the permitted set of variables and qualifies which variables are mandatory. Timeliness can be ascertained from the most recent batch of case registration dates, and uniqueness can be addressed by ensuring that the common data-set template does not lead to duplication of data contained in another variable. The more intricate quality dimensions regard integrity, accuracy, consistency, and data-completeness (completeness of the cancer cases within the catchment area of the population).

Whereas integrity and consistency can be assessed from the data, accuracy and data-completeness have to be ascertained from the real-life situation [35]. It is a process followed by CRs when cross checking summary values against data from the primary data feeds (e.g. hospital/clinical records). There may also be accuracy issues within the primary records themselves, such as incorrect data entry, which may be difficult to ascertain at the CR level. Integrity and consistency checks may be able to serve as a proxy in some instances where data entry is incorrect and in violation of the data rules; more subtle, systematic errors could possibly be detected using variances in frequency measures on variables. Establishing a formal data-quality process such as ISO 8000-8 at the first point of data capture is however perhaps the only way in which to assess the steps taken to ensure data accuracy. Such a process if harmonized across the data sources could provide a standard metric to integrate into the quality stamp of further processing operations. Metrics for estimating data completeness of CR data have been summarized in [37]. The data-quality dimensions most relevant to each stage of the CR data throughput chain are depicted in **Figure 1**.

The decision processes underlying the choices to combine data sets dependent on their quality metrics will depend largely on the intended purpose of the end application. The means for one possible decision-making framework is proposed in [38]. The framework is presented in terms of business-related data but raises a number of important considerations. It lays down five requirements for data-quality metrics and argues these requirements in practical examples of metrics proposed by others for measuring the specific quality dimensions of timeliness, completeness, reliability, correctness, and consistency (where correctness corresponds to accuracy and the metric for consistency can be applied also to integrity). The five requirements are:

1. provision of minimum and maximum values;

2. provision of interval-scaled values;

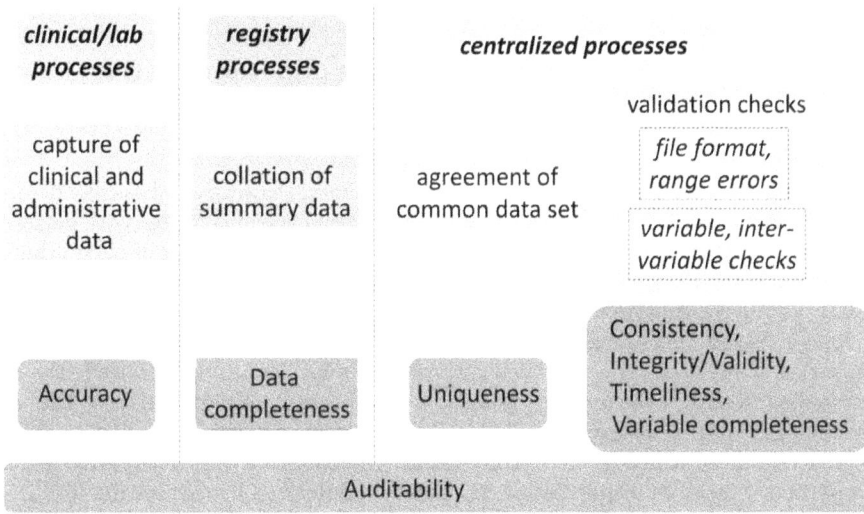

Figure 1.
Data-quality dimensions relevant to the different stages in the CR common data set throughput process. Auditability can span all processes.

3. means of determining the metric values on the basis of the associated configuration parameters and also whether the quality-criteria objectivity, reliability, and validity of the metric are fulfilled;

4. consistent aggregation of metric values on different data-view levels; and

5. economic efficiency of the metric (i.e. the cost incurred by the metric).

3. Ontologies and underlying foundations on description logics

Ontologies are relevant for describing the semantic relationships between entities in a data model. Bioportal [39] provides a comprehensive repository of biomedical ontologies. The Web Ontology Language (OWL) [40] underlies many of these ontologies and represents the concept definitions and relations between them as sets of Resource Description Framework (RDF) [41] graphs.

Interestingly however, ontologies formulated on description logic (such as OWL) can also be made to provide a basis for ascertaining the quality of data sets. A single tool can thereby be developed to handle both the semantic and the data-quality contexts. Whereas we present a model for achieving this for CR data, the concept is sufficiently generic to be applied to other data domains. An important requirement is that some form of data-validation rules are specified a priori.

For the purposes of comparing CR data, a common data set specifies the metadata of a minimum set variables to be included. Whereas, the availability of a common data set is not necessarily an essential aspect of the data-quality model, it does however aid the process to provide data-quality metrics easily interpretable by the end application.

3.1 Description logics

Description logics (DLs) are a family of languages used to represent in a structured and formal sense knowledge about a given domain [42]. They also provide the means for a degree of machine-reasoning allowing automated inferences to be made on the basis of statements concerning that knowledge.

DL languages are classified by language expressivity. Expressivity basically determines the richness of the modeling capacity of the language; a language with greater expressivity is able to model more complex relationships but at a cost of computing performance. In view of the latter, it is generally preferable to limit the DL expressivity to the minimum needed for the modeled aspects of the domain.

Knowledge about a domain can be captured in an OWL ontology using DL statements that are be classified into TBox and ABox axioms. TBox axioms refer to the terminological part of the ontology and ABox axioms, to the assertional part. The terminological part is analogous to the database concept of a database schema, which describes the structure or layout of the database while the assertional part is analogous to a particular instance or population of a database described by that schema [43]. Thus, OWL TBox axioms describe the hierarchies and relationships between OWL classes and ABox axioms describe specific instances of classes, also referred to as individuals.

The primary two semantic constructs DLs use are: unitary predicates (or concepts) describing entities equating to OWL classes/individuals; and binary predicates (or roles, equating to OWL properties) that describe relationships between entities. DLs are termed as decidable fragments of first-order logic [42] and TBox and ABox statements can in fact be expressed as first-order logic statements. The expressivity of a DL language determines the set of operators permitted. The Attributive Language with Complement (ALC) expressivity allows quite a rich modeling language to handle most of the validation checks in the ENCR common data set. ALC includes: subclasses ($\sqsubseteq$), intersections ($\sqcap$), unions ($\sqcup$), negation ($\neg$), existential restrictions ($\exists$), and universal restrictions ($\forall$). The restriction operators are used for qualifying the entities on which a given role acts, with $\exists$ specifying the notion of an "at-least-one relationship" and $\forall$ the notion of an "only relationship" and are similar to the existential and universal quantifiers of first-order logic.

3.2 Transcribing the data model and validation rules in DL

The data-validation rules encapsulate the part of the domain model that minimally needs to be modeled. The challenge lies in designing the ontology in a way that is straightforward to understand, easy to maintain, and models the data relationships satisfactorily whilst performing efficiently under automatic reasoning. Consideration should also be given to its potential reuse and extensibility. In practice, the interplay between all these factors may lead to a number of compromises.

Protégé [44] is a convenient, free, and open-source ontology-editing tool that provides a friendly user interface for creating and testing axioms. Such editing tools are particularly useful for aiding the design process in which the most appropriate design patterns may not be immediately obvious. Taking the example of the ICD-O-3 [45] spindle cell sarcoma with morphology code 8801 and tumor behavior code 3 (malignant behavior), the compound code (morphology-behavior) can be modeled in the ontology in several ways (where the morphology code has been prepended with the letter "M_" for more convenient class-naming purposes):

$$M\_8801\_3 \sqsubseteq M\_8801 \sqcap BehaviorCode3 \qquad (1)$$

$$M\_8801\_3 \sqsubseteq M\_8801 \sqcap \exists hasBehaviour.BehaviorCode3 \qquad (2)$$

$$M\_8801 \sqcap BehaviorCode3 \sqsubseteq M\_8801\_3 \qquad (3)$$

Eqs. (1) and (2) are similar apart from the fact that behavior in Eq. (2) has been expressed in terms of an existential restriction. Behavior may not even need to be modeled at all and just left implicit in the name of the class (since the trailing digit denotes the behavior code). The choice ultimately depends on how the morphology-behavior class will be used in other classes. For instance, a prostate tumor can have ICD-O-3 topography code C619, morphology code 8801, and behavior code 3 and may be modeled in a similar fashion to Eqs. (1)–(3):

$$ProstateTumor \sqsubseteq C619 \sqcap M\_8801\_3 \qquad (4)$$

$$ProstateTumor \sqsubseteq \exists hasTopography.C619 \sqcap \exists hasMorphology.M\_8801\_3 \qquad (5)$$

$$C619 \sqcap M\_8801\_3 \sqsubseteq ProstateTumor \qquad (6)$$

It could also be modeled as an Abox axiom to denote that this is a specific instance of a more general prostate cancer class. It is not necessarily a simple choice since there are advantages and disadvantages to each approach. With Eq. (5) the concepts of topography and morphology can be declared disjoint (a topography is not a morphology), but then modeling a tumor type or signature (e.g. $\exists hasTumorSignature.ProstateTumor$) would hide the topography and morphology codes in two existential restrictions:

$$\exists hasTumorSignature.(\exists hasTopography.C619 \sqcap \exists hasMorphology.M\_8801\_3) \qquad (7)$$

and thereby makes it a harder task to access the code values without increasing the language expressivity (such as including inverse operations or complex role inclusion axioms or other rules). It would be even harder to access the behavior code had Eq. (2) been used owing to the chain of existential restriction. Eq. (6) results in automatic class subsumption of the conjunction $C619 \sqcap M\_8801\_3$ under the class *ProstateTumor* but can lead to higher processing costs than Eq. (4) [46].

Nevertheless, subsumption is a primary mechanism used by automatic reasoners to make inferences on a knowledge base and is perhaps the most critical factor to take into account in the design of an ontology that models validation rules predominantly using TBox axioms. OWL uses the open world assumption (OWA) in which the truth of a statement is unknown unless it is expressly known to be true/false – the philosophy being that there may always be extra information not yet declared in the knowledge base that has further bearing on the statement. The consequence is that an entity having topography C619 and morphology M_8801_3 would not be considered as a *ProstateTumor* using Eq. (4) for the reason that there may be other as-yet undisclosed information to describe it further. The work-around would be either to make an equivalence – which can lead to subtle unintended consequences in more complex expressions – or to use the form of Eq. (6), which Protégé refers to as a general concept inclusion (GCI). CGIs provide several benefits in the correct context [47].

Also relevant is the balance between pre- and post-coordination of the ontology [48] – in pre-coordination, all the relationships are explicitly declared a priori, whereas in post-coordination a reasoner is used to infer relationships between entities a posteriori. In addition, other types of rules can be incorporated into OWL ontologies using the

Semantic Web Rule Language (SWRL). SWRL extends the expressivity of OWL DLs using Horn-like logic rules (in which logic statements are written in terms of an implication) and can overcome some limiting cases in OWL at the potential cost of decidability and interoperability [49]. **Table 4** summarizes some of the more important mechanisms that can be employed in validation-type tests.

There are thus a number of careful choices to be made dependent upon how the ontology will be used. The consequence of these design decisions may compromise the ability to reuse existing ontologies as well as render the ontology developed unsuitable for wider purposes.

3.3 Data shapes languages

An alternative to using an ontology for data validation, but which still draws directly from the data model, is to use a data shapes language such as the Shapes Constraint Language (SHACL) [50] or Shapes Expressions (ShEx) [51]. Both languages benefit from the possibility of formulating the rules under the closed world assumption (CWA) which, contrary to the OWA, considers a statement to be false unless it has otherwise explicitly been declared to be true.

The degree of complexity that can be handled for the inter-variable validation checks is more limited, but in cases where this does not pose a problem, SHACL in particular provides a number of advantages. SHACL is specifically intended as a

Pre/post coord	Mechanism	Utilization	Advantages/disadvantages
Post	Subsumption	Defined classes (TBox)	Ensures subsumption (since classes are equivalent). Can give rise to unintended equivalences
Post	Subsumption	General Concept Inclusions (TBox)	Ensures subsumption if the ontology design is correct. Needs careful ontology design to ensure the specific order of subsumption, which may conflict with other requirements
Post	Subsumption	Individuals and higher DL expressivities (ABox)	Greater flexibility and functionality. More difficult to control logic, and computationally expensive
Post	Inconsistency of class structure	Disjoint class definitions	Straightforward to catch any validation errors. Can lead to unintended class inconsistencies for ontologies with many class inter-relations
Post	Additional logic (internal to ontology)	SWRL	Provides extra functionality. Difficult to control if many rules and can lead to portability issues
Both	Additional logic (external to ontology)	Programming logic	Considerable control and extra functionality. Requires a dedicated computer program and extra maintenance
Pre	Comprehensive assertions	Predefinition of all entities and relationships	All the relationships are known a priori. Ontology can be very large and lead to performance issues if interfaced with ontologies requiring automatic reasoning

Table 4.
Summary of the most important ontology-based mechanisms that can used for data validation purposes with their main associated advantages/disadvantages.

Validation checks	Semantic Web tools	Quality dimensions measured
file format, range errors, less complex variable checks	Shape languages ShEx/SHACL	Integrity/Validity, Timeliness, Variable completeness
more complex variable checks, inter-variable checks, inter-record checks	OWL/ Description Logics, SWRL	Consistency, Integrity/Validity

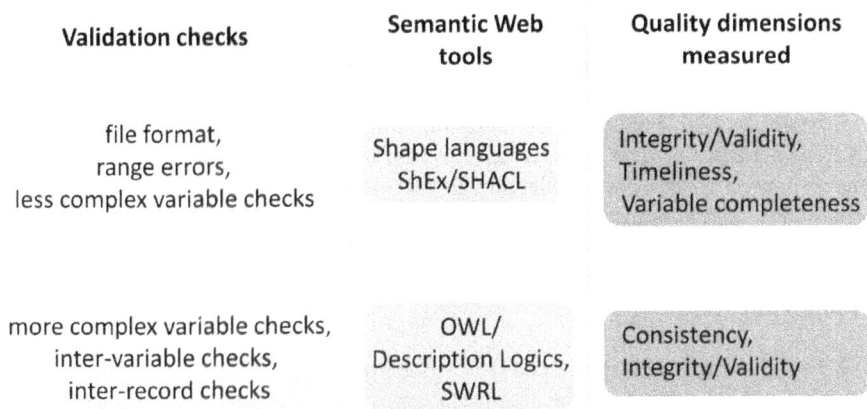

Figure 2.
Applicability of the semantic-web tools to the different steps of the validation process and the quality dimensions they are able to measure. Shape languages such as ShEx and SHACL provide the means for finding non-compliance to the more straightforward data validation rules. More complex validation checks require the increased functionality offered by DLs maybe in combination with SWRL and dedicated program logic.

language for describing constraints on RDF data and has been used to describe ontology design patterns for validating data in Electronic Health Records (EHRs) conforming to Clinical Information Modeling Initiative (CIMI) models [52].

ShEx can also be used to validate data but the underlying philosophy is different from that of SHACL. As noted in [53], ShEx is more grammar-related whilst SHACL is more constraint-related with the result that ShEx puts greater focus on validation results in contrast to SHACL that gives more attention to validation errors. As discussed in Section 4.4, ShEx is particularly useful in detecting syntactic and range errors in the preprocessing stages of CR data validation. **Figure 2** provides an overview of the applicability of the semantic-web tools to the different data-validation steps and the quality dimensions they are able to address.

4. Quality criteria for CR data

Before CR data can be compared at inter-regional or international level, they have to pass through a rigorous cleaning process. From the point of view statistical analysis, assessment of the quality and reliability of data hinges on the basic requirement of the representativeness of the data. A large CR data set for which reasonable doubts exist concerning the data representativeness has less value than a small CR data set with high representativeness.

More specifically for statistical analyses to derive incidence and survival indicators from CR data, the two required dimensions are completeness (the confidence that all diagnosed cancers in the population are actually included in the data set) and accuracy (the confidence that the proportion of cases with a given set of characteristics truly reflects reality [37, 54]). Whereas timeliness is another important dimension [54], it may lead to some trade-off with the degree of data completeness [55].

One cause of incompleteness observed in cancer survival studies results from the varying risk of death from other causes than cancer, and is more pronounced for the older age brackets [56] (competing-risks phenomenon). Other observational studies performed with the availability of additional, post factum data reveal that the level of incompleteness can also be cancer-site specific [55].

In addition, high-quality cancer data should have high comparability between different populations over time, which can best be achieved using up-to-date, homogeneous, and consistent data collection and recording procedures [54]. Application of the standard data validation rules is one way of ascertaining the comparability of data between different CRs, as discussed in the following sub-sections.

4.1 Inferring TNM stage

TNM (Tumor, Nodes, Metastases) is a globally recognized cancer staging classification system for describing the extent and spread of solid tumors in terms of tumor size, invasion of lymph nodes, and presence of metastases. One of the validation checks relates to the validity of TNM stage on the basis of the associated TNM parameters (including: topography, morphology, pathological/clinical T, N, and M codes, TNM edition, as well as age, and grade for certain tumor sites). Validity can be ascertained using the automatic reasoner to infer the stage from the parameters and compare it with the value provided by the registry. Axioms to model stage can be defined along the lines of the example taken for stage I prostate cancer:

$$TNMEd7SiteProstate \sqcap \exists hasBehavior.BehaviorCode3 \sqcap \exists hasT.(T1 \sqcup T2a) \sqcap$$
$$\exists hasN.N0 \sqcap \exists hasM.M0 \sqsubseteq TNMStageI \tag{8}$$

in which:

$$\exists hasTopography.C619 \sqcap \exists hasMorphology.Carcinoma \sqsubseteq TNMSiteProstate \tag{9}$$

$$TNMEd7SiteProstate \sqcap \exists hasTNMEdition.TNMEd7 \sqsubseteq TNMEd7SiteProstate \tag{10}$$

and all the ICD-O-3 morphologies associated with carcinoma have the form similar to:

$$\exists hasMorphology.M\_8140 \sqsubseteq \exists hasMorphology.Adenocarcinoma \tag{11}$$

in which, for example:

$$Adenocarcinoma \sqsubseteq Carcinoma \tag{12}$$

The resulting subsumption process for a CR case record passed in with the values: topography C619, morphology 8140, TNM edition 7, and TNM parameters: T2a, N0, M0 would be the following:

a. morphology M_8140 is subsumed under the class *Carcinoma* from Eqs. (11) and (12);

b. topography C619 together with the subsumed morphology M_8140 under the class *Carcinoma*, are further subsumed under the class *TNMEd7SiteProstate* from Eqs. (9) and (10);

c. the subsumpton result of (b) together with the specified TNM parameters, are finally subsumed under the stage class *TNMStageI*.

The value of stage inferred by the reasoner can then be compared with the stage value provided with the CR case record in order to validate the record. Axioms described in this manner can be developed to provide a modular structure to model TNM stage for all editions of TNM.

4.2 Multiple primary tumors validation check

For the purpose of deriving cancer incidence indicators, it is important in patients with multiple cancer case records to distinguish between tumors that are linked with an existing case and those that are not. The latter are referred to as multiple primary tumors and they need to be validated.

An international set of rules provides the definition of multiple primary tumors [57]. Transcribing the rules into DL requires a higher expressivity owing to the need for ABox statements, inverse relationships, and qualified number restrictions. These requirements arise from the need to analyze the different permutations of the possible tumor pairings according to the rules. The latter can be transcribed as a set of TBox axioms which are used by the reasoner to test the dependencies of multiple tumor cases defined as a set of ABox axioms. TBox axioms take the form of constructs encapsulated in Eqs. (13)–(16) below (described in greater detail in [58]):

$$\exists hasMorphology.MorphGroupX \sqcap \exists hasMorphoplogy.MorphGroupXDep \\ \sqsubseteq DuplicateMorphologyGroup \tag{13}$$

Eq. (13) models the conjunction of two dependent morphology groups as a sub-class of the class depicting a duplicate morphology, according to one of the multiple primary tumor rules:

$$DuplicateMorphologyGroup \sqcap \exists hasMorphoplogy.ICDO3HematologicalMorphology \\ \sqsubseteq DuplicatePrimaryCondition \tag{14}$$

Eq. (14) models the conjunction of a previously-determined duplicate morphology with a hematological morphology type as a duplicate primary tumor condition, according to another of the multiple primary tumor rules.

$$\geq 2hasTopography.(C26 \sqcup C68 \sqcup C76) \sqsubseteq DuplicateTopographyGroup \tag{15}$$

Eq. (15) models the rule that if the two topographies of a tumor pairing are in any of the "other or ill-defined" topography groups or subgroups they are considered a duplicate topography group.

$$DuplicateMorphologyGroup \sqcap DuplicateTopographyGroup \sqsubseteq \\ DuplicatePrimaryCondition \tag{16}$$

Eq. (16) models a resulting duplicate primary tumor for the case of a duplicate morphology and a duplicate topography.

ABox axioms are built up using permutations of tumor morphologies and topographies, where a tumor is defined by the TBox axiom as the conjunction of one morphology and one topography:

$$ICDO3Tumor \equiv= 1\, hasMorphology.ICDO3Morphology \sqcap\, = 1\, hasTopography.ICDO3Topography$$

(17)

Accessing the morphologies from two tumor individuals to derive a morphology permutation can be performed using the ABox axiom:

$$p1\_tpM1 : \exists hasMorphology.(\exists hasMorphology^-.(p1\_t1)) \sqcap$$
$$\exists hasMorphology.(\exists hasMorphology^-.(p1\_t2))$$

(18)

where the name of the individual $p1\_tpM1$ refers to the first morphology permutation of the two individual tumors $p1\_t1$, and $p1\_t2$ of a given patient $p1$. Since the morphologies have already been assigned in the tumor ABox axioms according to the pattern of Eq. (17), their specific values can be extracted using the inverse relationships in Eq. (18). Similar axioms can be defined for the topography permutations.

ABox axioms for the tumor pairings (containing a morphology pairing and a topography pairing) can then be specified according to the template:

$$(p1\_tc1, p1\_tpM1) : \exists hasTumorPermutationMorphology \sqcap$$
$$(p1\_tc1, p1\_tpT1) : \exists hasTumorPermutationTopography$$

(19)

in which $p1\_tc1$ refers to the first tumor pairing for patient $p1$ and $p1\_tpM1$ and $p1\_tpT1$ refer to the first morphology pair and topography pair respectively.

The axioms can be constructed automatically from the input records since the cancer-case records have a patient identifier and a tumor identifier and therefore all the tumor-pairing permutations can be ascertained in a preprocessing step. On the basis of the TBox axioms, the reasoner classifies the ABox axioms under the class *DuplicatePrimaryCondition* for instances where the multiple-primary rules are violated.

4.3 Tumor signature validation check

The third batch of validation checks concerns the specificities of tumor types, particularly in relation to parameters including basis of diagnosis, grade, age at diagnosis, sex, and topography-morphology-behavior inter-dependencies. These checks concern many of the rule tables provided in [15] and are examples of rules that be modeled in a variety of ways as discussed in Section 3.2 and which ultimately can be related to the balance between pre- and post-coordination of classes [48].

A tumor type, which we refer to as a tumor signature, comprises a topography/set of topographies in association with a set of morphologies. The topographies and morphologies may additionally specify a number of restrictions on values of associated variables such as age of patient at diagnosis, sex, basis of diagnosis, grade, etc.

Pre-coordination allows the greatest control over the definition of tumor signatures since it allows each tumor signature at its most granular level to be defined independently. Consequently, the permissible ranges of values of all the dependent variables can be specified for each tumor signature individually. The drawback to this approach is that it would result in over 200,000 unique tumor-signature classes and could have implications on reasoning speeds of other ontologies that use them.

The design used by SNOMED CT [59] to handle all the possible clinical terminology class definitions is to create a number of general classes in a pre-coordinated way and capture the specializations of those classes either in equivalent classes or GCI expressions that would be determined in a post-coordinated way by means of the reasoner [48]. Emulating such a design would allow, for instance, the qualifying rule of age on a given morphology/set of morphologies to be expressed as a specialization. Taking as an example the morphology M_8970 (Hepablastoma) which has a qualifying rule for ages greater than five, the associated morphology class can be sub-classed from a data property such that:

$$M\_8970 \sqsubseteq \exists ageAtDiagnosis.\{\geq 6\} \tag{20}$$

The resulting subsumption for hepablastomas thereby provides a mechanism through which it can be ensured that all qualifying rules are respected in the data.

4.4 Data quality metric

Once the rules have been established in the ontology, the individual data records can be validated according to the various groups of tests (e.g. stage, multiple primaries, tumor signature, etc.). Of the seven generally agreed dimensions for data quality listed in Section 2.2, integrity, consistency, and variable-completeness of CR common data sets are ascertained in a relatively straightforward manner for each of the tests and scored in percentage terms of conforming records using the metric:

$$\left(1 - \frac{R_e}{R_T}\right) \times 100 \tag{21}$$

where R_e is the total number of non-conforming records to the particular test parameters and R_T is the total number of records used within the test. Eq. (21) takes a similar form to that proposed in [60] for both completeness and consistency quality dimensions and was assessed in [38] to fulfill all the five data-metric requirements discussed in Section 2.2.1.

Variable-completeness would describe the extent of the availability of information/variables necessary for running the specific test. Integrity would provide information on the number of records passing the test. Consistency would then be a measure of data conformity across tests – e.g. consistency of the morphology-topography code combinations not just within one individual test but across all tests (TNM, multiple primary and tumor signature).

The syntactic part of the integrity dimension (as differentiated in ISO 8000-8) can be measured from a preprocessing stage which in general is necessary to ensure the correct format of the cancer-case records before passing them into the DL-based validation checks. This preprocessing stage can itself be performed also with direct reference to the data model using a shape language such as ShEx as discussed in Section 3.3. ShEx is particularly appropriate for validating the format and ranges of the variable values and benefits from the possibility of formulating the rules under the closed world assumption. The output of this stage can therefore provide a metric for data-type integrity also in percentage terms of records conforming to the ShEx schema.

As noted in Section 2.2.1, the quality dimensions posing greatest difficulty are data-completeness and accuracy. Various metrics to estimate the former have been proposed [37] and those based on mortality-incidence ratios or survival probabilities conform well to the data-metric requirements of [38]. Whereas accuracy issues may be insinuated from the result of the integrity/validity checks, the surest way of detecting them would be through a data-auditing process such as that advocated by ISO 8000-8.

4.5 Process automation

The chain of processes from preparation of the CR common data set to reading cancer case records into the ontology and performing the validation checks and counting the non-conforming records can be automated using the OWL application program interface (OWL-API) [61]. The OWL-API provides methods for accessing the ontology axioms, invoking the reasoner, and polling the results of the reasoning process. The API also allows the incorporation of program logic to permit greater expressivity although at the expense of increased maintenance.

The strength of the ontological approach is that the data model and the data-quality model – at least for the integrity and consistency dimensions remain in synchronization owing to the fact that they are integrated in the same sets of ontologies. Not only does this aid transparency of the validation process but it also simplifies maintenance and version control via the URIs pointing to the most current version of the ontology.

Moreover, the outputs of the validation process are readily verifiable by a trusted third party since it would basically be a matter of rerunning the checks on the CR file and comparing the outputs. For situations where the integrity of the quality metrics is important, the trusted third party can provide such assurance by integrating the validation checks together with the tests for data completeness and accuracy into a data-quality certification scheme such as ISO 8000-8.

5. Constructing a data-quality context

The quality context is as important as the semantic context for interoperability of CR data and as applicable to machine-based reasoning as it is to human-based reasoning; even though the semantics might admit the apparent compatibility of data sets, any inferences drawn from their combination could be legitimately challenged without due attention to the data quality. The importance of taking CR data completeness into consideration when comparing survival estimates between different populations has been emphasized previously [62]. In short, data quality is a critical issue for health data where erroneous inferences could lead to potentially dire consequences [63]. Encapsulating quality metrics in the metadata associated with the data set would adapt well to the FAIR digital object framework, and indeed such a model was proposed as far back as 1999 [64] and more recently in [65].

Agreeing a common set of data-quality metrics is however not an easy task and perhaps explains the lack of an overall framework. Whereas the difficulties are more acute for unstructured data [66] and require complicated semantic enrichment techniques [66], processes dealing with structured data pose less difficulty. The key to a potentially elegant solution able to unify both semantic and quality aspects of interoperability may lie in the use of OWL ontologies for describing common data models, or at least relevant parts of them.

If designed carefully, OWL axioms can be used for validating CR data sets against predefined rules as discussed in Section 4, thereby providing a quantitative quality index or set of indices for certain quality dimensions on which to base pragmatic decisions regarding the compatibility/comparability of different data sets. The availability of such a decision framework is critical to any eventual devolution of the centralized data-cleaning processes to the local level. It is also critical for purposes of secondary-data usage where the end user/application has to be aware of issues limiting the extent and purpose for which different data sets can be used.

With respect to the generally agreed seven quality dimensions, completeness of the mandatory variable set (variable-completeness), integrity and consistency are ascertainable from the validation process of the CR common data sets with each dimension being measured in percentage terms of conforming records as suggested in [35] and according to Eq. (21). Uniqueness can be ensured by a correct definition of the common data set template and therefore be provided as a default measure for all CR common data sets. Timeliness can be determined directly from the data set variable relating to cancer-case registration date providing a metric easy to measure. Data-completeness can be estimated in several ways as discussed in [37], one of which also provides a quantifiable metric along the lines of Eq. (21). The metrics for these quality dimensions would therefore all fulfill the requirements stipulated for a data metric supporting a decision-based framework [38].

The remaining quality dimension, accuracy, is dependent on the primary-data capture process, which is outside the control of cancer registries. Whereas, performance of the validation checks and frequency analyses of selected variables may provide some proxy measures for systematic errors, a more robust method would

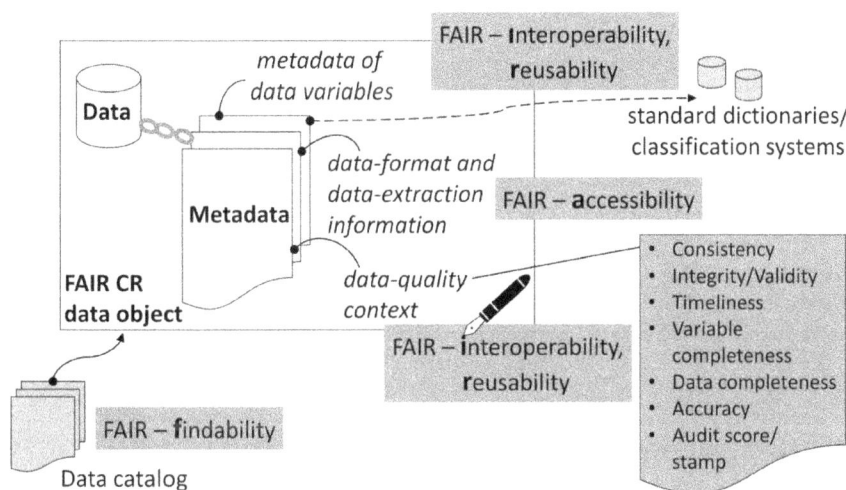

Figure 3.
Depiction of a FAIR cancer-registry data set in terms of a FAIR digital object (FDO). The FDO comprises the data itself and an associated set of metadata components that describe the data and their context. The FDO is registered in a catalog to make it findable. One of the metadata components provides information on how to access the data. Another metadata component describes the metadata and semantics of the data-set variables and links to standard dictionaries using the semantic relations of knowledge organization systems (e.g. SKOS). The semantic context provides an essential part of data interoperability and reusability. A further metadata component provides the data-quality context and "dots the 'i' of interoperability" by adding the second vital ingredient towards making the data interoperable and reusable.

need a data-auditing process in the various stages of the data pipeline. The resulting accuracy metrics could then be passed along through each stage to form a compound accuracy measure on the data set.

In this way, a comprehensive and structured data-quality context could be constructed and thereafter provided as an additional component of the associated FAIR digital object, as illustrated in **Figure 3**. This component would provide a direct means for decision-based mechanisms to compute quantitative differences between quality measures of data sets and thereby infer the suitability of their integration in some fashion.

6. Conclusions

Achieving data interoperability, at least in the widest sense, is a major challenge. In order to be able to integrate or compare heterogeneous data sets, data users non-expert in the respective data domains need a considerable amount of contextual information. Whereas these needs can be met partially by semantic linkage of meta-data, the aspect of data quality is crucial especially in quality-critical disciplines such as health. The FAIR data principles acknowledge the importance of data quality but do not address it directly.

A means of quantifying the data quality context in CR data sets along a number of representative and widely accepted quality dimensions has been presented. These metrics provide a quality context that can serve as an additional set of metadata within the associated FAIR digital object and made available with any aggregated data derived from it. The latter is an important consideration for entities having access only to the aggregated data sets for which the information is no longer available to verify the data quality directly from the validation rules themselves.

Having access to this type of data-quality information, even if measured in relatively simple terms, would enable data-processing entities to make certain informed decisions on the likely compatibility with other data sets. Not only is this a fundamental prerequisite to being able ultimately to federate the CR data-harmonization processes themselves but also to promoting the availability of CR data in ways that would prove useful and informative for secondary-data purposes. It would also allow more scrutiny and transparency on the results of secondary analyses that may have potentially far-reaching consequences.

Although the focus has been on CR data, the ideas are sufficiently generic to apply as a general framework to other data domains and is amenable to formalization in a data-quality auditing process such as ISO 8000-8 by providing a conceptual model and the defined means of verification against the model.

Acknowledgements

All the work was performed solely by the authors and there was also no grant finding to acknowledge. All authors are employed by governmental or supranational entities and report no additional funding for the development of this manuscript.

Conflict of interest

The authors declare that they have no competing interests.

Author details

Nicholas Nicholson*, Francesco Giusti, Luciana Neamtiu, Giorgia Randi,
Tadeusz Dyba, Manola Bettio, Raquel Negrao Carvalho, Nadya Dimitrova,
Manuela Flego and Carmen Martos
European Commission Joint Research Centre, Ispra, Italy

*Address all correspondence to: nicholas.nicholson@ec.europa.eu

IntechOpen

References

[1] Parkin DM. The evolution of the population-based cancer registry. Nature Reviews. Cancer. 2006;**6**:603-612. DOI: 10.1038/nrc1948

[2] Parkin DM. The role of cancer registries in cancer control. International Journal of Clinical Oncology. 2008;**13**: 102-111. DOI: 10.1007/s10147-008-0762-6

[3] dos Santos Silva I. Cancer Epidemiology: Principles and Methods, Ch 17. Lyon, France: IARC Press; 1999. 442 p. Available from: https://publications.iarc.fr/Non-Series-Publications/Other-Non-Series-Publications/Cancer-Epidemiology-Principles-And-Methods-1999

[4] Bray F, Znaor A, Cueva P, et al. Planning and Developing Population-Based Cancer Registration in Low- and Middle-Income Settings. 2014. Available from: https://www.who.int/immuniza tion/hpv/iarc_technical_report_no43.pdf [Accessed: July 26, 2021]

[5] Public Health Scotland. Scottish Cancer Registry – How Data are Collected. Available from: https://www. isdscotland.org/Health-Topics/Cancer/Scottish-Cancer-Registry/How-data-are-collected/ [Accessed: July 26, 2021]

[6] Tucker TC, Durbin EB, McDowell JK, Huang B. Unlocking the potential of population-based cancer registries. Cancer. 2019;**125**:3729-3737. DOI: 10.1002/cncr.32355

[7] Thompson CA, Jin A, Luft HS, Lichtensztajn DY, Allen L, Liang SY, et al. Population-based registry linkages to improve validity of electronic health record-based cancer research. Cancer Epidemiology, Biomarkers & Prevention. 2020;**29**(4):796-806. DOI: 10.1158/1055-9965.EPI-19-0882

[8] NIH Eunice Kennedy Shriver National Institute of Child Health and Human Development. Data Harmonization. Available from: https://www.icpsr.umich.edu/icpsrweb/content/DSDR/harmonization.html [Accessed: July 26, 2021]

[9] Arndt V, Holleczek B, Kajüter H, Luttmann S, Nennecke A, Zeissig SR, et al. Data from population-based cancer registration for secondary data analysis: Methodological challenges and perspectives. Das Gesundheitswesen. 2020;**82**(Suppl. 1):S62-S71. DOI: 10.25646/6907

[10] Antonio AS, Ferlay J, Soerjomataram I, Znaor A, Jemal A, Bray F. Bladder cancer incidence and mortality: A global overview and recent trends. European Urology. 2017;**71**(1): 96-108

[11] National Cancer Institute. North American Surveillance, Epidemiology, and End Results (SEER) Program. Available from: https://seer.cancer.gov/ [Accessed: July 26, 2021]

[12] European Commission. European Cancer Information System (ECIS). Available from: https://ecis.jrc.ec.europa. eu/ [Accessed: July 26, 2021]

[13] International Agency for Research on Cancer. Cancer Incidence in Five Continents (CI5). Available from: https://ci5.iarc.fr/Default.aspx [Accessed: July 26, 2021]

[14] International Agency for Research on Cancer. Global Cancer Observatory. Available from: https://gco.iarc.fr/ [Accessed: July 26, 2021]

[15] Martos C, Crocetti E, Visser O, Rous B, Giusti F, et al. A proposal on cancer

data quality checks: one common procedure for European cancer registries. JRC Technical Report, version 1.1. Luxembourg: Publications office of the European Union; 2018. 99 p. DOI: 10.2760/429053

[16] Wilkinson M, Dumontier M, Aalbersberg I, et al. The FAIR guiding principles for scientific data management and stewardship. Scientific Data. 2016;**3**: 160018. DOI: 10.1038/sdata.2016.18

[17] European Commission Expert Group on FAIR Data. European Commission Directorate General for Research and Innovation. Turning FAIR Into Reality. Luxembourg: Publications office of the European Union; 2018. 76 p. DOI: 10.2777/1524

[18] IDC. The Secondary Use of Health Data and Data-driven Innovation in the European Healthcare Industry. 2020. Available from: https://datalandscape.eu/sites/default/files/report/D3.6_Data-driven_Innovation_in_Health_21.01.2020_Final.pdf [Accessed: July 26, 2021]

[19] European Commission. European Health Data Space. Available from: ec.europa.eu/health/ehealth/dataspace_en [Accessed: July 26, 2021]

[20] W3C. Data Catalog Vocabulary (DCAT) – Version 2 Recommendation. 2020. Available from: https://www.w3.org/TR/vocab-dcat-2/ [Accessed: July 9, 2021]

[21] ISO/IEC. Information Technology – Metadata Registries (MDR). Part 1: Framework. 2015. Available from: https://www.iso.org/standard/61932.html [Accessed: July 9, 2021]

[22] W3C. SKOS Simple Knowledge Organization System. Available from: https://www.w3.org/2004/02/skos/ [Accessed: July 9, 2021]

[23] Fiume M, Cupak M, Keenan S, et al. Federated discovery and sharing of genomic data using Beacons. Nature Biotechnology. 2019;**37**:220-224. DOI: 10.1038/s41587-019-0046-x10.1038/s41587-019-0046-x

[24] Global Alliance for Genomics and Health. GA4GH Genome Beacons. Available from: https://beacon-project.io/categories/howto.html [Accessed: July 9, 2021]

[25] Sinaci AA, Laleci Erturkmen GB. A federated semantic metadata registry framework for enabling interoperability across clinical research and care domains. Journal of Biomedical Informatics. 2013;**46**:784-794. DOI: 10.1016/j.jbi.2013.05.009

[26] Nicholson N, Perego A. Interoperability of population-based patient registries. Journal of Biomedical Informatics. 2020;**112s**:100074. DOI: 10.1016/j.yjbinx.2020.100074

[27] MOLGENIS Data Platform. Available from: https://www.molgenis.org/ [Accessed: July 9, 2021]

[28] Apache Atlas. Available from: https://atlas.apache.org/#/ [Accessed: July 9, 2021]

[29] Corcho O, Eriksson M, Kurowski K, Ojsteršek M, Choirat C, van de Sanden Mark, Coppens F. EOSC interoperability framework - Report from the EOSC Executive Board Working Groups FAIR and Architecture. Luxembourg: Publications office of the European Union; 2021. 60 p. DOI:10.2777/620649

[30] Bonino da Silva Santos LO. FAIR Digital Object Framework Documentation Working Draft; Leiden: GO FAIR Foundation; 2021. Available from: https://fairdigitalobjectframework.org/ [Accessed: July 9, 2021]

[31] De Smedt K, Koureas D, Wittenburg P. FAIR digital objects for science: From data pieces to actionable knowledge units. Publica. 2020;8(2):21. DOI: 10.3390/publications8020021

[32] Data Interoperability Standards Consortium. Available from: https://datainteroperability.org/ [Accessed: July 9, 2021]

[33] GO FAIR. What FAIR is Not … . Available from: https://www.go-fair.org/resources/faq/what-fair-is-not/ [Accessed: July 9, 2021]

[34] Cai L, Zhu Y. The challenges of data quality and data quality assessment in the big data era. Data Science Journal. 2015;14:2. DOI: 10.5334/dsj-2015-002

[35] DAMA UK. The Six Primary Dimensions For Data Quality Assessment. Bristol: DAMA UK; 2013. Available from: https://docplayer.net/3987248-The-six-primary-dimensions-for-data-quality-assessment.html [Accessed: July 9, 2021]

[36] ISO. Data Quality – Part 8: Information and Data Quality: Concepts and Measuring ISO 8000-8. Geneva, Switzerland: ISO; 2015

[37] Parkin DM, Bray F. Evaluation of data quality in the cancer registry: Principles and methods Part II. Completeness. European Journal of Cancer. 2009;45(5):756-764

[38] Heinrich B, Hristova D, Klier M, Schiller A, Szubartowicz M. Requirements for data quality metrics. Journal of Data and Information Quality. 2018;9(2):1-32. DOI: 10.1145/3148238

[39] National Center for Biomedical Ontology. Bioportal. Available from: https://bioportal.bioontology.org/ [Accessed: July 9, 2021]

[40] W3C. Web Ontology Language (OWL). Available from: https://www.w3.org/OWL/ [Accessed: July 9, 2021]

[41] W3C. Resource Description Framework (RDF). Available from: https://www.w3.org/RDF/ [Accessed: July 9, 2021]

[42] Knorr M, Hitzler P. Description logics. In: Siekmann JH, editor. Handbook of the History of Logic. Vol. 9. The Netherlands: Elsevier Radarweg, AE Amsterdam; The Netherlands; 2014. pp. 659-678. DOI: 10.1016/B978-0-444-51624-4.50015-0

[43] Baader F, Horrocks I, Lutz C, Sattler U. An Introduction to Description Logic, Ch 1. Cambridge, UK: Cambridge University Press; 2017

[44] Protégé. A Free, Open-Source Ontology Editor and Framework for Building Intelligent Systems. Available from: https://protege.stanford.edu/ [Accessed: July 9, 2021]

[45] World Health Organization. International Classification of Diseases for Oncology (ICD-O) – 3rd Edition, 1st Revision. 2013. Available from: https://apps.who.int/iris/handle/10665/96612 [Accessed: July 26, 2021]

[46] Hammar K. Reasoning performance indicators for ontology design patterns. In: Proceedings of the 4th International Conference on Ontology and Semantic Web Patterns (WOP'13); Aachen, Germany: CEUR-WS; 2013. pp. 27–38

[47] Sattler U, Stevens R. Being complex on the left-hand-side: General Concept Inclusions. Ontogenesis. 2012. Available from: http://ontogenesis.knowledgeblog.org/1288 [Accessed: July 9, 2021]

[48] Stevens R, Sattler U. Post-coordination: Making things up as you go

along. Ontogenesis. 2013. Available from: http://ontogenesis.knowledgeblog. org/1305 [Accessed: July 9, 2021]

[49] W3C. SWRL: A Semantic Web Rule Language Combining OWL and RuleML. Available from: https://www.w3.org/Sub mission/SWRL/ [Accessed: July 9, 2021]

[50] W3C. Shapes Constraint Language (SHACL). Available from: https://www. w3.org/TR/shacl/ [Accessed: July 9, 2021]

[51] W3C. Shape Expressions Language (ShEx). Available from: http://shex.io/ shex-semantics/ [Accessed: July 9, 2021]

[52] Martínez-Costa C, Schulz S. Validating EHR clinical models using ontology patterns. Journal of Biomedical Informatics. 2017;**76**:124-137. DOI: 10.1016/j.jbi.2017.11.001

[53] Labra Gayo JE, Prud'hommeaux E, Boneva I, Kontokostas D. Validating RDF Data. In: Ding Y, Groth P, series editors. Synthesis Lectures on Semantic Web: Theory and Technology, Lecture #16. San Rafael, California, USA: Morgan & Claypool Publishers; 2018. 304 p. DOI: 10.2200/ S00786ED1V01Y201707WBE016

[54] Bray F, Parkin DM. Evaluation of data quality in the cancer registry: Principles and methods. Part I: Comparability, validity and timeliness. European Journal of Cancer. 2009;**45**(5): 747-755

[55] Zanetti R, Schmidtmann I, Sacchetto L, Binder-Foucard F, Bordoni A, Coza D, et al. Completeness and timeliness: Cancer registries could/ should improve their performance. European Journal of Cancer. 2015;**51**(9): 1091-1098

[56] Schuster NA, Hoogendijk EO, Kok AAL, Twisk JWR, Heymans MW.

Ignoring competing events in the analysis of survival data may lead to biased results: A nonmathematical illustration of competing risk analysis. Journal of Clinical Epidemiology. 2020; **122**:42-48. DOI: 10.1016/j. jclinepi.2020.03.004

[57] International Association of Cancer Registries. International rules for multiple primary cancers. Asian Pacific Journal of Cancer Prevention. 2005;**6**(1): 104-106

[58] Nicholson NC, Giusti F, Bettio M, Negrao Carvalho R, Dimitrova N, Dyba T, et al. An ontology to model the international rules for multiple primary malignant tumours in cancer registration. Applied Sciences. 2021;**11**: 7233. DOI: 10.3390/app11167233

[59] SNOMED CT. Available from: http:// www.snomed.org [Accessed: July 9, 2021]

[60] Blake R, Mangiameli P. The effects and interactions of data quality and problem complexity on classification. Journal of Data and Information Quality. 2011;**2**(2):1-28. DOI: 10.1145/ 1891879.1891881

[61] Horridge M, Bechhofer S. The OWL API: A java API for OWL ontologies. Semantic Web. 2011;**2**(1):11-21. DOI: 10.3233/SW-2011-0025

[62] Robinson D, Sankila R, Hakulinen T, Moller H. Interpreting international comparisons of cancer survival: The effects of incomplete registration and the presence of death certificate only cases on survival estimates. European Journal of Cancer. 2007;**43**:909-913

[63] The Connecting for Health Common Framework. Background Issues on Data Quality. 2006. Available from: http:// bok.ahima.org/PdfView?oid=63654 [Accessed: July 14, 2021]

[64] Vassiliadis P, Bouzeghoub M, Quix C. Towards Quality-Oriented Data Warehouse Usage and Evolution. In: Advanced Information Systems Engineering, 11th International Conference (CAiSE'99); 14-18 June 1999; Berlin, Heidelberg, Germany: Springer-Verlag; 1999. p. 164-179. DOI: 10.1.1.42.6458

[65] European Commission Directorate-General for Informatics. Data Quality Management. 2019. Available from: https://joinup.ec.europa.eu/sites/default/files/document/2019-09/SEMIC [Accessed: July 9, 2021]

[66] Cichy C, Rass S. An overview of data quality frameworks. IEEE Access. 2019; 7:24634-24648. DOI: 10.1109/ACCESS.2019.2899751

www.ingramcontent.com/pod-product-compliance
Lightning Source LLC
Chambersburg PA
CBHW081600190326
41458CB00015B/5661